CONTENTS

BREAKFAST RECIPES

1. Sweet Potato Chickpeas Hash

Servings: 4
Cooking Time: 30 Minutes
Ingredients:
- 14.5 oz can chickpeas, drained
- 1 tsp paprika
- 1 tsp garlic powder
- 1 sweet potato, peeled and cubed
- 1 tbsp olive oil
- 1 bell pepper, chopped
- 1 onion, diced
- 1/2 tsp ground black pepper
- 1 tsp salt

Directions:
1. Fit the oven with the rack in position
2. Spread sweet potato, chickpeas, bell pepper, and onion in a baking pan.
3. Drizzle with oil and season with paprika, garlic powder, pepper, and salt. Stir well.
4. Set to bake at 390 F for 35 minutes, after 5 minutes, place the baking pan in the oven.

Nutrition Info: Calories 203 Fat 4.9 g Carbohydrates 34.9 g Sugar 4.7 g Protein 6.5 g Cholesterol 0 mg

2. Latkes

Servings: 5
Cooking Time: 7 Minutes
Ingredients:
- 1 large onion
- 5 large potatoes peeled
- 4 large eggs
- ¼ cup potato starch
- 2 tsp kosher salt
- ½ tsp baking powder
- Olive oil

Directions:
1. Scrub your potatoes well and place them in a food processor. Besides, place the shredded potatoes in a bowl of cool water and set it aside.
2. Rinse the food in the processor and grate the onions. Place your grated onions in a paper towel and squeeze out the liquid.
3. In a medium sized bowl whisk your eggs and add matzo, pepper, 1 tsp potato starch, baking powder and grated onion. Drain the water from the potatoes and save the starch that remains in your bowl.
4. Scoop the starch from the potato bowl and add to the latke mixture. Form latkes from the mixture in flat circles and dip into dry potato starch. Add oil and place them in an air fryer

5. Air fry your latkes at 360-degree Fahrenheit for 8 minutes
6. and turn in the middle once it indicates turn food.
7. Serve while hot.
Nutrition Info: Calories 68 Fat 4g, Carbohydrates 6g, Protein 2g.

3. Cheesy Hash Brown Cups

Servings: 6
Cooking Time: 9 Minutes
Ingredients:
- 4 eggs, beaten
- 2¼ cups frozen hash browns, thawed
- 1 cup diced ham
- ½ cup shredded Cheddar cheese
- ½ teaspoon Cajun seasoning
- Cooking spray

Directions:
1. Lightly spritz a 12-cup muffin tin with cooking spray.
2. Combine the beaten eggs, hash browns, diced ham, cheese, and Cajun seasoning in a medium bowl and stir until well blended.
3. Spoon a heaping 1½ tablespoons of egg mixture into each muffin cup.
4. Put the muffin tin into Rack Position 1, select Convection Bake, set temperature to 350ºF (180ºC) and set time to 9 minutes.
5. When cooked, the muffins will be golden brown.
6. Allow to cool for 5 to 10 minutes on a wire rack and serve warm.

4. Cauliflower Hash Brown

Servings: 4
Cooking Time: 10 Minutes
Ingredients:
- 2 cups cauliflower, finely grated, soaked and drained
- 2 tablespoons xanthan gum
- Salt, to taste
- Pepper powder, to taste
- 2 teaspoons chili flakes
- 1 teaspoon garlic
- 1 teaspoon onion powder
- 2 teaspoons vegetable oil

Directions:
1. Preheat the Air fryer to 300-degree F and grease an Air fryer basket with oil.
2. Heat vegetable oil in a nonstick pan and add cauliflower.

3. Sauté for about 4 minutes and dish out the cauliflower in a plate.
4. Mix the cauliflower with xanthum gum, salt, chili flakes, garlic and onion powder.
5. Mix well and refrigerate the hash for about 20 minutes.
6. Place the hash in the Air fryer basket and cook for about 10 minutes.
7. Flip the hash after cooking halfway through and dish out to serve warm.
Nutrition Info: Calories: 291, Fat: 2.8g, Carbs: 6.5g, Sugar: 4.5g, Protein: 6.6g, Sodium: 62mg

5. Bourbon Vanilla French Toast

Servings: 4
Cooking Time: 6 Minutes
Ingredients:
- 2 large eggs
- 2 tablespoons water
- $^2/_3$ cup whole or 2% milk
- 1 tablespoon butter, melted
- 2 tablespoons bourbon
- 1 teaspoon vanilla extract
- 8 (1-inch-thick) French bread slices
- Cooking spray

Directions:
1. Spray the baking pan with cooking spray.
2. Beat the eggs with the water in a shallow bowl until combined. Add the milk, melted butter, bourbon, and vanilla and stir to mix well.
3. Dredge 4 slices of bread in the batter, turning to coat both sides evenly. Transfer the bread slices to the baking pan.
4. Slide the baking pan into Rack Position 1, select Convection Bake, set temperature to 320ºF (160ºC) and set time to 6 minutes.
5. Flip the slices halfway through the cooking time.
6. When cooking is complete, the bread slices should be nicely browned.
7. Remove from the oven to a plate and serve warm.

6. Spinach And Ricotta Pockets

Servings: 8 Pockets
Cooking Time: 10 Minutes
Ingredients:
- 2 large eggs, divided
- 1 tablespoon water
- 1 cup baby spinach, roughly chopped
- ¼ cup sun-dried tomatoes, finely chopped
- 1 cup ricotta cheese
- 1 cup basil, chopped
- ¼ teaspoon red pepper flakes
- ¼ teaspoon kosher salt
- 2 refrigerated rolled pie crusts
- 2 tablespoons sesame seeds

Directions:
1. Spritz the air fryer basket with cooking spray.
2. Whisk an egg with water in a small bowl.
3. Combine the spinach, tomatoes, the other egg, ricotta cheese, basil, red pepper flakes, and salt in a large bowl. Whisk to mix well.
4. Unfold the pie crusts on a clean work surface and slice each crust into 4 wedges. Scoop up 3 tablespoons of the spinach mixture on each crust and leave ½ inch space from edges.
5. Fold the crust wedges in half to wrap the filling and press the edges with a fork to seal.
6. Arrange the wraps in the pan and spritz with cooking spray. Sprinkle with sesame seeds.
7. Put the air fryer basket on the baking pan and slide into Rack Position 2, select Air Fry, set temperature to 380ºF (193ºC) and set time to 10 minutes.
8. Flip the wraps halfway through the cooking time.
9. When cooked, the wraps will be crispy and golden.
10. Serve immediately.

7. Prosciutto & Salami Egg Bake

Servings: 2
Cooking Time: 20 Minutes
Ingredients:
- 1 beef sausage, chopped
- 4 slices prosciutto, chopped
- 3 oz salami, chopped
- 1 cup grated mozzarella cheese
- 4 eggs, beaten
- ½ tsp onion powder

Directions:
1. Preheat on Bake function to 350 F. Whisk the eggs with the onion powder. Brown the sausage in a skillet over medium heat for 2 minutes. Remove to the egg mixture and add in mozzarella cheese, salami, and prosciutto and give it a stir. Pour the egg mixture in a greased baking pan and cook for 10-15 minutes until golden brown on top. Serve.

8. Corned Beef Hash With Eggs

Servings: 4
Cooking Time: 25 Minutes
Ingredients:
- 2 medium Yukon Gold potatoes, peeled and cut into ¼-inch cubes
- 1 medium onion, chopped
- $^1/_3$ cup diced red bell pepper

- 3 tablespoons vegetable oil
- ½ teaspoon dried thyme
- ½ teaspoon kosher salt, divided
- ½ teaspoon freshly ground black pepper, divided
- ¾ pound (340 g) corned beef, cut into ¼-inch pieces
- 4 large eggs

Directions:
1. In a large bowl, stir together the potatoes, onion, red pepper, vegetable oil, thyme, ¼ teaspoon of the salt and ¼ teaspoon of the pepper. Spread the vegetable mixture into the baking pan in an even layer.
2. Slide the baking pan into Rack Position 2, select Roast, set temperature to 375ºF (190ºC) and set time to 25 minutes.
3. After 15 minutes, remove the pan from the oven and add the corned beef. Stir the mixture to incorporate the corned beef. Return the pan to the oven and continue cooking.
4. After 5 minutes, remove the pan from the oven. Using a large spoon, create 4 circles in the hash to hold the eggs. Gently crack an egg into each circle. Season the eggs with the remaining ¼ teaspoon of the salt and ¼ teaspoon of the pepper. Return the pan to the oven. Continue cooking for 3 to 5 minutes, depending on how you like your eggs.
5. When cooking is complete, remove the pan from the oven. Serve immediately.

9. Breakfast Sandwich

Servings: 1
Cooking Time: 7minutes
Ingredients:
- 2 Bacon Slices
- 1 Egg
- 1 English muffin Salt& Pepper to taste

Directions:
1. Beat the egg into a soufflé cup and add salt and pepper to taste.
2. Heat the air fryer to 390°F and place the soufflé cup, English muffin and bacon into the tray.
3. Cook all the ingredients for 6-10 minutes. Assemble sandwich and enjoy.
Nutrition Info: Calories 113 Fat 8.2 g
Carbohydrates 0.3 g Sugar 0.2 g Protein 5.4 g
Cholesterol 18 mg

10. Italian Sandwich

Servings: 1
Cooking Time: 7 Minutes
Ingredients:

- 2 bread slices
- 4 tomato slices
- 4 mozzarella cheese slices
- 1 tbsp olive oil
- 1 tbsp fresh basil, chopped
- Salt and black pepper to taste

Directions:
1. Preheat Breville on Toast function to 350 F. Place the bread slices in the toaster oven and toast for 5 minutes. Arrange two tomato slices on each bread slice. Season with salt and pepper.
2. Top each slice with 2 mozzarella slices. Return to the oven and cook for 1 more minute. Drizzle the caprese toasts with olive oil and top with chopped basil.

11. Balsamic Chicken With Spinach & Kale

Servings: 1
Cooking Time: 20 Minutes
Ingredients:
- ½ cup baby spinach
- ½ cup romaine lettuce, shredded
- 3 large kale leaves, chopped
- 1 chicken breast, cut into cubes
- 2 tbsp olive oil
- 1 tsp balsamic vinegar
- 1 garlic clove, minced
- Salt and black pepper to taste

Directions:
1. Place the chicken, some olive oil, garlic, salt, and pepper in a bowl; toss to combine. Put on a lined baking dish and cook in the Breville for 14 minutes at 390F on Bake function.
2. Meanwhile, place the greens in a large bowl. Add the remaining olive oil and balsamic vinegar. Season with salt and pepper and toss to combine. Top with the sliced chicken and serve.

12. Vanilla Granola

Servings: 4
Cooking Time: 40 Minutes
Ingredients:
- 1 cup rolled oats
- 3 tablespoons maple syrup
- 1 tablespoon sunflower oil
- 1 tablespoon coconut sugar
- ¼ teaspoon vanilla
- ¼ teaspoon cinnamon
- ¼ teaspoon sea salt

Directions:
1. Mix together the oats, maple syrup, sunflower oil, coconut sugar, vanilla, cinnamon, and sea salt in a

medium bowl and stir to combine. Transfer the mixture to the baking pan.

2. Slide the baking pan into Rack Position 1, select Convection Bake, set temperature to 248ºF (120ºC) and set time to 40 minutes.
3. Stir the granola four times during cooking.
4. When cooking is complete, the granola will be mostly dry and lightly browned.
5. Let the granola stand for 5 to 10 minutes before serving.

13. Toasted Cinnamon Bananas

Servings: 1
Cooking Time: 10 Minutes
Ingredients:
*   1 ripe banana
*   Lemon juice
*   2 teaspoons honey
*   Ground cinnamon

Directions:
1. Start by preheating toaster oven to 350°F.
2. Slice bananas lengthwise and place them on a greased baking sheet.
3. Brush each slice with lemon juice.
4. Drizzle honey and sprinkle cinnamon over each slice.
5. Bake for 10 minutes.

Nutrition Info: Calories: 154, Sodium: 3 mg, Dietary Fiber: 4.2 g, Total Fat: 0.5 g, Total Carbs: 40.2 g, Protein: 1.5 g.

14. Golden Cod Tacos With Salsa

Servings: 4
Cooking Time: 15 Minutes
Ingredients:
*   2 eggs
*   1¼ cups Mexican beer
*   1½ cups coconut flour
*   1½ cups almond flour
*   ½ tablespoon chili powder
*   1 tablespoon cumin
*   Salt, to taste
*   1 pound (454 g) cod fillet, slice into large pieces
*   4 toasted corn tortillas
*   4 large lettuce leaves, chopped
*   ¼ cup salsa
*   Cooking spray

Directions:
1. Spritz the air fryer basket with cooking spray.
2. Break the eggs in a bowl, then pour in the beer. Whisk to combine well.

3. Combine the coconut flour, almond flour, chili powder, cumin, and salt in a separate bowl. Stir to mix well.
4. Dunk the cod pieces in the egg mixture, then shake the excess off and dredge into the flour mixture to coat well. Arrange the cod in the pan.
5. Put the air fryer basket on the baking pan and slide into Rack Position 2, select Air Fry, set temperature to 375ºF (190ºC) and set time to 15 minutes.
6. Flip the cod halfway through the cooking time.
7. When cooking is complete, the cod should be golden brown.
8. Unwrap the toasted tortillas on a large plate, then divide the cod and lettuce leaves on top. Baste with salsa and wrap to serve.

15. Cinnamon & Vanilla Toast

Servings: 6
Cooking Time: 10 Minutes
Ingredients:
*   12 bread slices
*   ½ cup sugar
*   1 ½ tsp cinnamon
*   1 stick of butter, softened
*   1 tsp vanilla extract

Directions:
1. Preheat Breville on Toast function to 300 F. Combine all ingredients, except the bread, in a bowl. Spread the buttery cinnamon mixture onto the bread slices. Place the bread slices in the oven and press Start. Cook for 8 minutes. Serve.

16. Peanut Butter And Jelly Banana Boats

Servings: 1
Cooking Time: 15 Minutes
Ingredients:
*   1 banana
*   1/4 cup peanut butter
*   1/4 cup jelly
*   1 tablespoon granola

Directions:
1. Start by preheating toaster oven to 350°F.
2. Slice banana lengthwise and separate slightly.
3. Spread peanut butter and jelly in the gap.
4. Sprinkle granola over the entire banana.
5. Bake for 15 minutes.

Nutrition Info: Calories: 724, Sodium: 327 mg, Dietary Fiber: 9.2 g, Total Fat: 36.6 g, Total Carbs: 102.9 g, Protein: 20.0 g.

17. Avocado And Zucchini Mix

Servings: 4
Cooking Time: 15 Minutes
Ingredients:
- 2 avocados, peeled, pitted and roughly cubed
- 2 zucchinis, roughly cubed
- 1 tablespoon olive oil
- 2 spring onions, chopped
- 8 eggs, whisked
- 1 teaspoon sweet paprika
- A pinch of salt and black pepper
- 1 tablespoon dill, chopped

Directions:
1.   Heat up the air fryer with the oil at 350 degrees F, add the zucchinis and the spring onions and cook for 2 minutes.
2.   Add the avocados and the other ingredients, cook the mix for 13 minutes more, divide into bowls and serve.

Nutrition Info: calories 232, fat 12, fiber 2, carbs 10, protein 5

18. Apple-cinnamon Empanadas

Servings: 2-4
Cooking Time: 30 Minutes
Ingredients:
- 2-3 baking apples, peeled & diced
- 2 tsp.s of cinnamon
- 1/4 cup white sugar
- 1 tablespoon brown sugar
- 1 tablespoon of water
- 1/2 tablespoon cornstarch
- ¼ tsp. of vanilla extract
- 2 tablespoons of margarine or margarine
- 4 pre-made empanada dough shells (Goya)

Directions:
1.   In a bowl, add together white sugar, brown sugar, cornstarch and cinnamon; set aside. Put the diced apples in a pot and place on a stovetop.
2.   Add the combined dry ingredients to the apples, then add the water, vanilla extract, and margarine; stirring well to mix.
3.   Cover pot and cook on high heat. Once it starts boiling, lower heat and simmer, until the apples are soft. Remove from the heat and cool.
4.   Lay the empanada shells on a clean counter. Ladle the apple mixture into each of the shells, being careful to prevent spillage over the edges. Fold shells to fully cover apple mixture, seal edges with water, pressing down to secure with a fork.
5.   Cover the air fryer basket with tin foil but leave the edges uncovered so that air can circulate through the basket. Place the empanadas shells in the foil lined air fryer basket, set temperature at 350°F and timer for 15 minutes.
6.   Halfway through, slide the frying basket out and flip the empanadas using a spatula. Remove when golden, and serve directly from the basket onto plates.

Nutrition Info: Calories 113 Fat 8.2 g Carbohydrates 0.3 g Sugar 0.2 g Protein 5.4 g Cholesterol 18 mg

19. Avocado Oil Gluten Free Banana Bread Recipe

Ingredients:
- 1/2 cup Granulated Sugar
- 1 cup Mashed Banana
- 1/2 cup Light Brown Sugar
- 1/3 cup Avocado Oil, (or canola oil)
- 2 cups All-Purpose Gluten Free Flour, (see notes)
- 3/4 teaspoon Xanthan Gum, (omit if your flour blend contains it)
- 1 teaspoon Baking Powder
- 1/2 teaspoon Baking Soda
- 1/2 teaspoon Fine Sea Salt
- 2 large Eggs, room temperature
- 2/3 cup Milk, (dairy free or regular milk), room temperature
- 1 teaspoon Pure Vanilla Extract

Directions:
1.   Preheat oven to 350°F and spray a 9x9 inch square pan with non-stick spray and line with parchment paper.
2.   In a large bowl, whisk together the flour, xanthan gum, baking powder, baking soda, salt, and granulated sugar.
3.   In a separate bowl, whisk together the mashed banana, brown sugar, oil, eggs, milk, and vanilla extract. Pour the wet ingredients into the dry ingredients and stir to combine.
4.   Pour the batter into the prepared pan and bake at 350°F for 25-30 minutes or until a toothpick or cake tester comes out clean or with a few moist crumbs attached. Cooking time will vary depending on your oven - mine took 29 minutes.
5.   Cool the bread in the pan on a cooling rack. Cut into 16 pieces and serve slightly warm or room temperature.
6.   To store, wrap tightly in foil or store slices in an air-tight container. It will stay fresh up to 3 days. This bread also freezes well. To freeze, slice into individual pieces and freeze in a freezer bag.

20. Delicious Baked Eggs

Servings: 8

Cooking Time: 45 Minutes
Ingredients:
- 12 eggs
- 1/2 cup all-purpose flour
- 16 oz cottage cheese
- 16 oz cheddar cheese, shredded
- 1 tsp salt

Directions:
1. Fit the oven with the rack in position
2. Grease 9*13-inch baking pan with butter and set aside.
3. In a large bowl, whisk eggs with flour, cottage cheese, cheddar cheese, and salt.
4. Pour egg mixture into the prepared baking pan.
5. Set to bake at 350 F for 50 minutes. After 5 minutes place the baking pan in the preheated oven.
6. Serve and enjoy.

Nutrition Info: Calories 402 Fat 26.5 g Carbohydrates 9.3 g Sugar 1 g Protein 31 g Cholesterol 310 mg

21. Sausage Omelet

Servings: 2
Cooking Time: 13 Minutes
Ingredients:
- 4 eggs
- 1 bacon slice, chopped
- 2 sausages, chopped
- 1 yellow onion, chopped

Directions:
1. In a bowl, crack the eggs and beat well.
2. Add the remaining ingredients and gently, stir to combine.
3. Place the mixture into a baking pan.
4. Press "Power Button" of Air Fry Oven and turn the dial to select the "Air Fry" mode.
5. Press the Time button and again turn the dial to set the cooking time to 13 minutes.
6. Now push the Temp button and rotate the dial to set the temperature at 320 degrees F.
7. Press "Start/Pause" button to start.
8. When the unit beeps to show that it is preheated, open the lid.
9. Arrange pan over the "Wire Rack" and insert in the oven.
10. Cut into equal-sized wedges and serve hot.

Nutrition Info: Calories 325 Total Fat 23.1 g Saturated Fat 7.4 g Cholesterol 368 mg Sodium 678 mg Total Carbs 6 g Fiber 1.2 g Sugar 3 g Protein 22.7 g

22. Zucchini Breakfast Bread

Servings: 10
Cooking Time: 50 Minutes

Ingredients:
- 2 eggs
- 1 1/2 cups zucchini, grated
- 1 tsp vanilla extract
- 1/4 cup yogurt
- 1/2 tsp baking powder
- 1 1/2 cups whole wheat flour
- 1/2 cup applesauce
- 1/4 cup coconut sugar
- 1 tsp ground cinnamon
- 1/2 tsp baking soda
- 1/2 cup apple, grated
- 1/4 tsp sea salt

Directions:
1. Fit the oven with the rack in position
2. In a bowl, mix all dry ingredients.
3. In another bowl, whisk eggs, coconut sugar, vanilla, yogurt, and applesauce.
4. Add dry ingredients mixture into the wet mixture and stir until well combined.
5. Add apples and zucchini and stir well.
6. Pour batter into the 9*5-inch greased loaf pan.
7. Set to bake at 350 F for 55 minutes, after 5 minutes, place the loaf pan in the oven.
8. Slice and serve.

Nutrition Info: Calories 103 Fat 1.2 g Carbohydrates 19.1 g Sugar 3.3 g Protein 3.7 g Cholesterol 33 mg

23. Parsley Sausage Patties

Servings: 4
Cooking Time: 20 Minutes
Ingredients:
- 1 lb ground Italian sausage
- ¼ cup breadcrumbs
- 1 tsp dried parsley
- 1 tsp red pepper flakes
- Salt and black pepper to taste
- ¼ tsp garlic powder
- 1 egg, beaten

Directions:
1. Preheat Breville on Bake function to 350 F. Line a baking sheet with parchment paper. Combine all the ingredients in a large bowl.
2. Make patties out of the sausage mixture and arrange them on the baking sheet. Press Start. Cook for 15 minutes until golden.

24. Pork Momos

Servings: 4
Cooking Time: 20 Minutes
Ingredients:
- 2 tablespoons olive oil
- 1 pound (454 g) ground pork

- 1 shredded carrot
- 1 onion, chopped
- 1 teaspoon soy sauce
- 16 wonton wrappers
- Salt and ground black pepper, to taste
- Cooking spray

Directions:
1.   Heat the olive oil in a nonstick skillet over medium heat until shimmering.
2.   Add the ground pork, carrot, onion, soy sauce, salt, and ground black pepper and sauté for 10 minutes or until the pork is well browned and carrots are tender.
3.   Unfold the wrappers on a clean work surface, then divide the cooked pork and vegetables on the wrappers. Fold the edges around the filling to form momos. Nip the top to seal the momos.
4.   Arrange the momos in the air fryer basket and spritz with cooking spray.
5.   Put the air fryer basket on the baking pan and slide into Rack Position 2, select Air Fry, set temperature to 320ºF (160ºC) and set time to 10 minutes.
6.   When cooking is complete, the wrappers will be lightly browned.
7.   Serve immediately.

25.   Spicy Apple Turnovers

Servings: 4
Cooking Time: 20 Minutes
Ingredients:
- 1 cup diced apple
- 1 tablespoon brown sugar
- 1 teaspoon freshly squeezed lemon juice
- 1 teaspoon all-purpose flour, plus more for dusting
- ¼ teaspoon cinnamon
- ⅛ teaspoon allspice
- ½ package frozen puff pastry, thawed
- 1 large egg, beaten
- 2 teaspoons granulated sugar

Directions:
1.   Whisk together the apple, brown sugar, lemon juice, flour, cinnamon and allspice in a medium bowl.
2.   On a clean work surface, lightly dust with the flour and lay the puff pastry sheet. Using a rolling pin, gently roll the dough to smooth out the folds, seal any tears and form it into a square. Cut the dough into four squares.
3.   Spoon a quarter of the apple mixture into the center of each puff pastry square and spread it evenly in a triangle shape over half the pastry, leaving a border of about ½ inch around the edges of the pastry. Fold the pastry diagonally over the filling to form triangles. With a fork, crimp the edges to seal

them. Place the turnovers in the baking pan, spacing them evenly.
4.   Cut two or three small slits in the top of each turnover. Brush with the egg. Sprinkle evenly with the granulated sugar.
5.   Slide the baking pan into Rack Position 1, select Convection Bake, set temperature to 350ºF (180ºC) and set time to 20 minutes.
6.   When cooking is complete, remove the pan from the oven. The turnovers should be golden brown and the filling bubbling. Let cool for about 10 minutes before serving.

26.   Pea And Potato Samosas With Chutney

Servings: 16 Samosas
Cooking Time: 22 Minutes
Ingredients:
- Dough:
- 4 cups all-purpose flour, plus more for flouring the work surface
- ¼ cup plain yogurt
- ½ cup cold unsalted butter, cut into cubes
- 2 teaspoons kosher salt
- 1 cup ice water
- Filling:
- 2 tablespoons vegetable oil
- 1 onion, diced
- 1½ teaspoons coriander
- 1½ teaspoons cumin
- 1 clove garlic, minced
- 1 teaspoon turmeric
- 1 teaspoon kosher salt
- ½ cup peas, thawed if frozen
- 2 cups mashed potatoes
- 2 tablespoons yogurt
- Cooking spray
- Chutney:
- 1 cup mint leaves, lightly packed
- 2 cups cilantro leaves, lightly packed
- 1 green chile pepper, deseeded and minced
- ½ cup minced onion
- Juice of 1 lime
- 1 teaspoon granulated sugar
- 1 teaspoon kosher salt
- 2 tablespoons vegetable oil

Directions:
1.   Put the flour, yogurt, butter, and salt in a food processor. Pulse to combine until grainy. Pour in the water and pulse until a smooth and firm dough forms.
2.   Transfer the dough on a clean and lightly floured working surface. Knead the dough and shape it into a ball. Cut in half and flatten the halves into 2 discs.

Wrap them in plastic and let sit in refrigerator until ready to use.

3. Meanwhile, make the filling: Heat the vegetable oil in a saucepan over medium heat.
4. Add the onion and sauté for 5 minutes or until lightly browned.
5. Add the coriander, cumin, garlic, turmeric, and salt and sauté for 2 minutes or until fragrant.
6. Add the peas, potatoes, and yogurt and stir to combine well. Turn off the heat and allow to cool.
7. Meanwhile, combine the ingredients for the chutney in a food processor. Pulse to mix well until glossy. Pour the chutney in a bowl and refrigerate until ready to use.
8. Make the samosas: Remove the dough discs from the refrigerator and cut each disc into 8 parts. Shape each part into a ball, then roll the ball into a 6-inch circle. Cut the circle in half and roll each half into a cone.
9. Scoop up 2 tablespoons of the filling into the cone, press the edges of the cone to seal and form into a triangle. Repeat with remaining dough and filling.
10. Spritz the air fryer basket with cooking spray. Arrange the samosas in the pan and spritz with cooking spray.
11. Put the air fryer basket on the baking pan and slide into Rack Position 2, select Air Fry, set temperature to 360ºF (182ºC) and set time to 15 minutes.
12. Flip the samosas halfway through the cooking time.
13. When cooked, the samosas will be golden brown and crispy.
14. Serve the samosas with the chutney.

27. Zucchini Breakfast Casserole

Servings: 8
Cooking Time: 50 Minutes
Ingredients:
- 12 eggs
- 2 small zucchinis, shredded
- 1 lb ground sausage
- 3 tomatoes, sliced
- 3 tbsp coconut flour
- 1/4 cup coconut milk
- 1/4 tsp pepper
- 1/2 tsp salt

Directions:
1. Fit the oven with the rack in position
2. Cook sausage in a pan until lightly brown.
3. Transfer sausage to a large mixing bowl.
4. Add coconut flour, milk, eggs, zucchini, pepper, and salt. Stir well.
5. Add eggs and whisk until well combined.

6. Pour bowl mixture into the greased casserole dish and top with tomato slices.
7. Set to bake at 350 F for 55 minutes, after 5 minutes, place the casserole dish in the oven.
8. Serve and enjoy.
Nutrition Info: Calories 330 Fat 25 g Carbohydrates 5.7 g Sugar 2.7 g Protein 20.8 g Cholesterol 293 mg

28. Cheddar Eggs With Potatoes

Servings: 3
Cooking Time: 24 Minutes
Ingredients:
- 3 potatoes, thinly sliced
- 2 eggs, beaten
- 2 oz cheddar cheese, shredded
- 1 tbsp all-purpose flour
- ½ cup coconut cream

Directions:
1. Preheat Breville on AirFry function to 390 F. Place the potatoes the basket and press Start. Cook for 12 minutes. Mix the eggs, coconut cream, and flour until the cream mixture thickens.
2. Remove the potatoes from the oven, line them in the ramekin and top with the cream mixture. Top with the cheddar cheese. Cook for 12 more minutes.

29. Rarebit Air-fried Egg

Servings: 2-4
Cooking Time: 5 Minutes
Ingredients:
- 4 Slices Sourdough
- 4 Eggs
- 1/3 cup ale
- 1 & 1/2 cups cheddar, grated
- 1 tsp. mustard powder
- 1/2 tsp. paprika
- Black Pepper to taste
- 2 tsp. Worcestershire Sauce

Directions:
1. Fry eggs, sunny side up and set to one side. Preheat Air Fryer to 350°F.
2. In a bowl, add together the cheddar, ale, paprika, mustard powder, and Worcestershire sauce.
3. Spread just one side of each slice of sourdough with the cheddar mixture.
4. Place the bread slices into the Air fryer tray. Cook for about 3 minutes until slightly browned.
5. Top the rarebits with fried eggs and spice with pepper to taste.
Nutrition Info: Calories 115 Fat 9.2 g Carbohydrates 0.3 g Sugar 0.3 g Protein 5.4 g Cholesterol 19 mg

30. Creamy Potato Gratin With Nutmeg

Servings: 4
Cooking Time: 30 Minutes
Ingredients:
- 1 lb potatoes, peeled and sliced
- ½ cup sour cream
- ½ cup mozzarella cheese, grated
- ½ cup milk
- ½ tsp nutmeg
- Salt and black pepper to taste

Directions:
1. Preheat Breville on Bake function to 390 F. In a bowl, combine sour cream, milk, pepper, salt, and nutmeg. Place the potato slices in the bowl with the milk mixture and stir to coat well.
2. Transfer the mixture to a baking dish and press Start. Cook for 20 minutes, then sprinkle grated cheese on top and cook for 5 more minutes. Serve warm.

31. Moist Orange Bread Loaf

Servings: 10
Cooking Time: 50 Minutes
Ingredients:
- 4 eggs
- 4 oz butter, softened
- 1 cup of orange juice
- 1 orange zest, grated
- 1 cup of sugar
- 2 tsp baking powder
- 2 cups all-purpose flour
- 1 tsp vanilla

Directions:
1. Fit the oven with the rack in position
2. In a large bowl, whisk eggs and sugar until creamy.
3. Whisk in vanilla, butter, orange juice, and orange zest.
4. Add flour and baking powder and mix until combined.
5. Pour batter into the greased 9*5-inch loaf pan.
6. Set to bake at 350 F for 55 minutes, after 5 minutes, place the loaf pan in the oven.
7. Slice and serve.
Nutrition Info: Calories 286 Fat 11.3 g Carbohydrates 42.5 g Sugar 22.4 g Protein 5.1 gCholesterol 90 mg

32. Thai Pork Sliders

Servings: 6 Sliders
Cooking Time: 14 Minutes
Ingredients:
- 1 pound (454 g) ground pork

- 1 tablespoon Thai curry paste
- 1½ tablespoons fish sauce
- ¼ cup thinly sliced scallions, white and green parts
- 2 tablespoons minced peeled fresh ginger
- 1 tablespoon light brown sugar
- 1 teaspoon ground black pepper
- 6 slider buns, split open lengthwise, warmed
- Cooking spray

Directions:
1. Spritz the air fryer basket with cooking spray.
2. Combine all the ingredients, except for the buns in a large bowl. Stir to mix well.
3. Divide and shape the mixture into six balls, then bash the balls into six 3-inch-diameter patties.
4. Arrange the patties in the basket and spritz with cooking spray.
5. Put the air fryer basket on the baking pan and slide into Rack Position 2, select Air Fry, set temperature to 375ºF (190ºC) and set time to 14 minutes.
6. Flip the patties halfway through the cooking time.
7. When cooked, the patties should be well browned.
8. Assemble the buns with patties to make the sliders and serve immediately.

33. Ham And Cheese Bagel Sandwiches

Servings: 2
Cooking Time: 5 Minutes
Ingredients:
- 2 bagels
- 4 teaspoons honey mustard
- 4 slices cooked honey ham
- 4 slices Swiss cheese

Directions:
1. Start by preheating toaster oven to 400°F.
2. Spread honey mustard on each half of the bagel.
3. Add ham and cheese and close the bagel.
4. Bake the sandwich until the cheese is fully melted, approximately 5 minutes.
Nutrition Info: Calories: 588, Sodium: 1450 mg, Dietary Fiber: 2.3 g, Total Fat: 20.1 g, Total Carbs: 62.9 g, Protein: 38.4 g.

34. Sweet Pineapple Oatmeal

Servings: 6
Cooking Time: 45 Minutes
Ingredients:
- 2 cups old-fashioned oats
- 1/2 cup coconut flakes
- 1 cup pineapple, crushed

- 2 eggs, lightly beaten
- 1/3 cup yogurt
- 1/3 cup butter, melted
- 1/2 tsp baking powder
- 1/3 cup brown sugar
- 1/2 tsp vanilla
- 2/3 cup milk
- 1/2 tsp salt

Directions:
1. Fit the oven with the rack in position
2. In a mixing bowl, mix together oats, baking powder, brown sugar, and salt.
3. In a separate bowl, beat eggs with vanilla, milk, yogurt, and butter.
4. Add egg mixture into the oat mixture and stir to combine.
5. Add coconut and pineapple and stir to combine.
6. Pour oat mixture into the greased 8-inch baking dish.
7. Set to bake at 350 F for 50 minutes, after 5 minutes, place the baking dish in the oven.
8. Serve and enjoy.

Nutrition Info: Calories 304 Fat 16.4 g Carbohydrates 33.2 g Sugar 13.6 g Protein 7.5 g Cholesterol 85 mg

35. Beef And Bell Pepper Fajitas

Servings: 4
Cooking Time: 10 Minutes
Ingredients:
- 1 pound (454 g) beef sirloin steak, cut into strips
- 2 shallots, sliced
- 1 orange bell pepper, sliced
- 1 red bell pepper, sliced
- 2 garlic cloves, minced
- 2 tablespoons Cajun seasoning
- 1 tablespoon paprika
- Salt and ground black pepper, to taste
- 4 corn tortillas
- ½ cup shredded Cheddar cheese
- Cooking spray

Directions:
1. Spritz the air fryer basket with cooking spray.
2. Combine all the ingredients, except for the tortillas and cheese, in a large bowl. Toss to coat well.
3. Pour the beef and vegetables in the pan and spritz with cooking spray.
4. Put the air fryer basket on the baking pan and slide into Rack Position 2, select Air Fry, set temperature to 360ºF (182ºC) and set time to 10 minutes.
5. Stir the beef and vegetables halfway through the cooking time.

6. When cooking is complete, the meat will be browned and the vegetables will be soft and lightly wilted.
7. Unfold the tortillas on a clean work surface and spread the cooked beef and vegetables on top. Scatter with cheese and fold to serve.

36. Herby Mushrooms With Vermouth

Servings: 4
Cooking Time: 20 Minutes
Ingredients:
- 2 lb portobello mushrooms, sliced
- 2 tbsp vermouth
- ½ tsp garlic powder
- 1 tbsp olive oil
- 2 tsp herbs
- 1 tbsp duck fat, softened

Directions:
1. Mix duck fat, garlic powder, and herbs in a bowl. Pour the mixture over the mushrooms and top with vermouth. Place the mushrooms in a baking dish and press Start. Cook for 15 minutes on Bake function at 350 F. Serve warm.

37. Fennel And Eggs Mix

Servings: 4
Cooking Time: 20 Minutes
Ingredients:
- 1 tablespoon avocado oil
- 1 yellow onion, chopped
- ½ teaspoon cumin, ground
- 1 teaspoon rosemary, dried
- 8 eggs, whisked
- 1 fennel bulb, shredded
- 1 tablespoon chives, chopped
- Salt and black pepper to the taste

Directions:
1. In a bowl, combine the onion with the eggs, fennel and the other ingredients except the oil and whisk.
2. Heat up your air fryer with the oil at 360 degrees F, add the oil, add the fennel mix, cover, cook for 20 minutes, divide between plates and serve for breakfast.

Nutrition Info: calories 220, fat 11, fiber 3, carbs 4, protein 6

38. Cheesy Potato & Spinach Frittata

Servings: 4
Cooking Time: 35 Minutes
Ingredients:
- 3 cups potato cubes, boiled

- 2 cups spinach, chopped
- 5 eggs, lightly beaten
- ¼ cup heavy cream
- 1 cup grated mozzarella cheese
- ½ cup parsley, chopped
- Fresh thyme, chopped
- Salt and black pepper to taste

Directions:
1. Spray the Air Fryer tray with oil. Arrange the potatoes inside.
2. In a bowl, whisk eggs, cream, spinach, mozzarella, parsley, thyme, salt and pepper, and pour over the potatoes. Cook in your for 16 minutes at 360 F on Bake function until nice and golden. Serve sliced.

39. Zucchini Fritters

Servings: 4
Cooking Time: 7 Minutes
Ingredients:
- 10½ ounces zucchini, grated and squeezed
- 7 ounces Halloumi cheese
- ¼ cup all-purpose flour
- 2 eggs
- 1 teaspoon fresh dill, minced
- Salt and black pepper, to taste

Directions:
1. Preheat the Air fryer to 360F and grease a baking dish.
2. Mix together all the ingredients in a large bowl.
3. Make small fritters from this mixture and place them on the prepared baking dish.
4. Transfer the dish in the Air Fryer basket and cook for about 7 minutes.
5. Dish out and serve warm.
Nutrition Info: Calories: 250 Cal Total Fat: 17.2 g Saturated Fat: 0 g Cholesterol: 0 mg Sodium: 330 mg Total Carbs: 10 g Fiber: 0 g Sugar: 2.7 g Protein: 15.2 g

40. Sausage And Cheese Quiche

Servings: 4
Cooking Time: 25 Minutes
Ingredients:
- 12 large eggs
- 1 cup heavy cream
- Salt and black pepper, to taste
- 12 ounces (340 g) sugar-free breakfast sausage
- 2 cups shredded Cheddar cheese
- Cooking spray

Directions:
1. Coat the baking pan with cooking spray.

2. Beat together the eggs, heavy cream, salt and pepper in a large bowl until creamy. Stir in the breakfast sausage and Cheddar cheese.
3. Pour the sausage mixture into the prepared pan.
4. Slide the baking pan into Rack Position 1, select Convection Bake, set temperature to 375ºF (190ºC) and set time to 25 minutes.
5. When done, the top of the quiche should be golden brown and the eggs will be set.
6. Remove from the oven and let sit for 5 to 10 minutes before serving.

41. Breakfast Oatmeal Cake

Servings: 8
Cooking Time: 25 Minutes
Ingredients:
- 2 eggs
- 1 tbsp coconut oil
- 3 tbsp yogurt
- 1/2 tsp baking powder
- 1 tsp cinnamon
- 1 tsp vanilla
- 3 tbsp honey
- 1/2 tsp baking soda
- 1 apple, peel & chopped
- 1 cup oats

Directions:
1. Fit the oven with the rack in position
2. Line baking dish with parchment paper and set aside.
3. Add 3/4 cup oats and remaining ingredients into the blender and blend until smooth.
4. Add remaining oats and stir well.
5. Pour mixture into the prepared baking dish.
6. Set to bake at 350 F for 30 minutes. After 5 minutes place the baking dish in the preheated oven.
7. Slice and serve.
Nutrition Info: Calories 114 Fat 3.6 g Carbohydrates 18.2 g Sugar 10 g Protein 3.2 g Cholesterol 41 mg

42. Potato Egg Casserole

Servings: 6
Cooking Time: 35 Minutes
Ingredients:
- 5 eggs
- 2 medium potatoes, cut into 1/2-inch cubes
- 1 green bell pepper, diced
- 1 small onion, chopped
- 1 tbsp olive oil
- 1/2 cup cheddar cheese, shredded
- 3/4 tsp pepper
- 3/4 tsp salt

Directions:

1. Fit the oven with the rack in position
2. Spray 9*9-inch casserole dish with cooking spray and set aside.
3. Heat oil in a pan over medium heat.
4. Add onion and sauté for 1 minute. Add potatoes, bell peppers, 1/2 tsp pepper, and 1/2 tsp salt and sauté for 4 minutes.
5. Transfer sautéed vegetables to the prepared casserole dish and spread evenly.
6. In a bowl, whisk eggs with remaining pepper and salt.
7. Pour egg mixture over sautéed vegetables in a casserole dish. Sprinkle cheese on top.
8. Set to bake at 350 F for 40 minutes. After 5 minutes place the casserole dish in the preheated oven.
9. Serve and enjoy.
Nutrition Info: Calories 171 Fat 9.2 g Carbohydrates 14.3 g Sugar 2.6 g Protein 8.5 g Cholesterol 146 mg

43. Feta & Tomato Tart With Olives

Servings: 2
Cooking Time: 40 Minutes
Ingredients:
- 4 eggs
- ½ cup tomatoes, chopped
- 1 cup feta cheese, crumbled
- 1 tbsp fresh basil, chopped
- 1 tbsp fresh oregano, chopped
- ¼ cup Kalamata olives, pitted and chopped
- ¼ cup onions, chopped
- 2 tbsp olive oil
- ½ cup milk
- Salt and black pepper to taste

Directions:
1. Preheat Breville on Bake function to 340 F. Brush a pie pan with olive oil. Beat the eggs along with the milk, salt, and pepper. Stir in the remaining ingredients. Pour the egg mixture into the pan and press Start. Cook for 15-18 minutes. Serve sliced.

44. Quick Cheddar Omelet

Servings: 1
Cooking Time: 15 Minutes
Ingredients:
- 2 eggs, beaten
- 1 cup cheddar cheese, shredded
- 1 whole onion, chopped
- 2 tbsp soy sauce

Directions:
1. Preheat Breville on AirFry function to 340 F. Drizzle soy sauce over the chopped onions. Sauté the onions ina greased pan over medium heat for 5 minutes; turn off the heat.
2. In a bowl, mix the eggs with salt and pepper. Pour the egg mixture over onions and cook in the Breville for 6 minutes. Top with cheddar cheese and bake for 4 more minutes. Serve and enjoy!

45. Prawn And Cabbage Egg Rolls Wraps

Servings: 4
Cooking Time: 18 Minutes
Ingredients:
- 2 tablespoons olive oil
- 1 carrot, cut into strips
- 1-inch piece fresh ginger, grated
- 1 tablespoon minced garlic
- 2 tablespoons soy sauce
- ¼ cup chicken broth
- 1 tablespoon sugar
- 1 cup shredded Napa cabbage
- 1 tablespoon sesame oil
- 8 cooked prawns, minced
- 8 egg roll wrappers
- 1 egg, beaten
- Cooking spray

Directions:
1. Spritz the air fryer basket with cooking spray. Set aside.
2. Heat the olive oil in a nonstick skillet over medium heat until shimmering.
3. Add the carrot, ginger, and garlic and sauté for 2 minutes or until fragrant.
4. Pour in the soy sauce, broth, and sugar. Bring to a boil. Keep stirring.
5. Add the cabbage and simmer for 4 minutes or until the cabbage is tender.
6. Turn off the heat and mix in the sesame oil. Let sit for 15 minutes.
7. Use a strainer to remove the vegetables from the liquid, then combine with the minced prawns.
8. Unfold the egg roll wrappers on a clean work surface, then divide the prawn mixture in the center of wrappers.
9. Dab the edges of a wrapper with the beaten egg, then fold a corner over the filling and tuck the corner under the filling. Fold the left and right corner into the center. Roll the wrapper up and press to seal. Repeat with remaining wrappers.
10. Arrange the wrappers in the pan and spritz with cooking spray.
11. Put the air fryer basket on the baking pan and slide into Rack Position 2, select Air Fry, set temperature to 370ºF (188ºC) and set time to 12 minutes.
12. Flip the wrappers halfway through the cooking time.

13. When cooking is complete, the wrappers should be golden.
14. Serve immediately.

46. Whole-wheat Muffins With Blueberries

Servings: 8 Muffins
Cooking Time: 25 Minutes
Ingredients:
- ½ cup unsweetened applesauce
- ½ cup plant-based milk
- ½ cup maple syrup
- 1 teaspoon vanilla extract
- 2 cups whole-wheat flour
- ½ teaspoon baking soda
- 1 cup blueberries
- Cooking spray

Directions:
1. Spritz a 8-cup muffin pan with cooking spray.
2. In a large bowl, stir together the applesauce, milk, maple syrup and vanilla extract. Whisk in the flour and baking soda until no dry flour is left and the batter is smooth. Gently mix in the blueberries until they are evenly distributed throughout the batter.
3. Spoon the batter into the muffin cups, three-quarters full.
4. Put the muffin pan into Rack Position 1, select Convection Bake, set temperature to 375ºF (190ºC) and set time to 25 minutes.
5. When cooking is complete, remove from the oven and check the muffins. You can stick a knife into the center of a muffin and it should come out clean.
6. Let rest for 5 minutes before serving.

47. Almond & Cinnamon Berry Oat Bars

Servings: 10
Cooking Time: 40 Minutes
Ingredients:
- 3 cups rolled oats
- ½ cup ground almonds
- ½ cup flour
- 1 tsp baking powder
- 1 tsp ground cinnamon
- 3 eggs, lightly beaten
- ½ cup canola oil
- ⅓ cup milk
- 2 tsp vanilla extract
- 2 cups mixed berries

Directions:
1. Spray the baking pan with cooking spray. In a bowl, add oats, almonds, flour, baking powder and cinnamon into and stir well. In another bowl, whisk eggs, oil, milk, and vanilla.

2. Stir the wet ingredients gently into the oat mixture. Fold in the berries. Pour the mixture in the pan and place in the toaster oven. Cook for 15-20 minutes at 350 F on Bake function until is nice and soft. Let cool and cut into bars to serve.

48. Hearty Sweet Potato Baked Oatmeal

Servings: 6
Cooking Time: 30 Minutes
Ingredients:
- 1 egg, lightly beaten
- 1 tsp vanilla
- 1 1/2 cups milk
- 1 tsp baking powder
- 2 tbsp ground flax seed
- 1 cup sweet potato puree
- 1/4 tsp nutmeg
- 2 tsp cinnamon
- 1/3 cup maple syrup
- 2 cups old fashioned oats
- 1/4 tsp salt

Directions:
1. Fit the oven with the rack in position
2. Spray an 8-inch square baking pan with cooking spray and set aside.
3. Add all ingredients except oats into the mixing bowl and mix until well combined.
4. Add oats and stir until just combined.
5. Pour mixture into the prepared baking pan.
6. Set to bake at 350 F for 35 minutes. After 5 minutes place the baking pan in the preheated oven.
7. Serve and enjoy.
Nutrition Info: Calories 355 Fat 6.3 g Carbohydrates 62.3 g Sugar 17.1 g Protein 10.9 g Cholesterol 32 mg

49. Fried Apple Lemon & Vanilla Turnovers

Ingredients:
- 2 sheets frozen puff pastry
- (17-ounce/480g package), thawed (keep
- cold until use)
- 3 medium Granny Smith apples, peeled
- and diced (about 3 cups)
- 2 tablespoons (30g) unsalted butter
- L cup (70g) dark brown sugar
- 1 teaspoon vanilla extract
- 1 teaspoon lemon juice
- ¾ teaspoon ground cinnamon
- ¼ teaspoon kosher salt
- 1 egg
- 1 tablespoon water
- Turbinado sugar for sprinkling

Directions:

1. Combine filling ingredients in a medium saucepan and cook over medium heat, stirring occasionally, until apples are tender and syrup is thick, about 10 minutes.
2. Transfer apple mixture to a plate and chill in the refrigerator until cool to the touch, about 20 minutes.
3. Scramble egg and water in a small bowl.
4. Place 1 sheet of puff pastry on a clean cutting board; reserve second sheet in the refrigerator.
5. Divide pastry into 4 equal squares. Spoon 2 tablespoons apple mixture onto the center of each square.
6. Brush the edges of each square with egg wash. Fold pastry diagonally over apple mixture and seal the edges with a fork.
7. Place turnovers on a plate and refrigerate while preparing remaining turnovers. Repeat steps 4 to 6 with second sheet of puff pastry.
8. Select AIRFRY/325°F (165°C)/SUPER CONVECTION/20 minutes and press START to preheat oven.
9. Place turnovers on air fry rack. Brush tops with egg wash and sprinkle with turbinado sugar. Make 3 small slits in each turnover.
10. Cook in rack position 4 until puffed and golden brown, about 20 minutes. Serve warm or at room temperature.

50. Cheesy Eggs With Fried Potatoes

Servings: 4
Cooking Time: 30 Minutes
Ingredients:
- 2 lb potatoes, thinly sliced
- 1 tbsp olive oil
- 2 eggs, beaten
- 2 oz cheddar cheese, grated
- 1 tbsp all-purpose flour
- ½ cup coconut cream
- Salt and black pepper to taste

Directions:
1. Season the potatoes with salt and pepper and place them in the Air Fryer basket; drizzle with olive oil. Fit in the baking tray and cook for 12 minutes at 350 F on Air Fry function.
2. Mix the eggs, coconut cream, and flour in a bowl until the cream mixture thickens. Remove the potatoes from the fryer oven, line them in a baking pan and top with the cream mixture. Sprinkle with cheddar cheese. Cook for 12 more minutes. Serve warm.

51. Asparagus And Cheese Strata

Servings: 4
Cooking Time: 17 Minutes

Ingredients:
- 6 asparagus spears, cut into 2-inch pieces
- 1 tablespoon water
- 2 slices whole-wheat bread, cut into ½-inch cubes
- 4 eggs
- 3 tablespoons whole milk
- 2 tablespoons chopped flat-leaf parsley
- ½ cup grated Havarti or Swiss cheese
- Pinch salt
- Freshly ground black pepper, to taste
- Cooking spray

Directions:
1. Add the asparagus spears and 1 tablespoon of water in the baking pan.
2. Slide the baking pan into Rack Position 1, select Convection Bake, set temperature to 330ºF (166ºC) and set time to 4 minutes.
3. When cooking is complete, the asparagus spears will be crisp-tender.
4. Remove the asparagus from the pan and drain on paper towels.
5. Spritz the pan with cooking spray. Place the bread and asparagus in the pan.
6. Whisk together the eggs and milk in a medium mixing bowl until creamy. Fold in the parsley, cheese, salt, and pepper and stir to combine. Pour this mixture into the baking pan.
7. Select Bake and set time to 13 minutes. Put the pan back to the oven. When done, the eggs will be set and the top will be lightly browned.
8. Let cool for 5 minutes before slicing and serving.

52. Ham Shirred Eggs With Parmesan

Servings: 2
Cooking Time: 20 Minutes
Ingredients:
- 4 eggs
- 2 tbsp heavy cream
- 4 ham slices
- 3 tbsp Parmesan cheese, shredded
- ¼ tsp paprika
- Salt and black pepper to taste
- 2 tsp chives, chopped

Directions:
1. Preheat Breville on AirFry function to 320 F. Arrange the ham slices on the bottom of a greased pan to cover it completely. Whisk 1 egg along with the heavy cream, salt, and pepper in a bowl.
2. Pour the mixture over the ham slices. Crack the other eggs on top. Sprinkle with Parmesan cheese and press Start. Cook for 14 minutes. Sprinkle with paprika and chives and serve.

53. Baked Avocado With Eggs

Servings: 2
Cooking Time: 9 Minutes
Ingredients:
- 1 large avocado, halved and pitted
- 2 large eggs
- 2 tomato slices, divided
- ½ cup nonfat Cottage cheese, divided
- ½ teaspoon fresh cilantro, for garnish

Directions:
1. Line the baking pan with aluminium foil.
2. Slice a thin piece from the bottom of each avocado half so they sit flat. Remove a small amount from each avocado half to make a bigger hole to hold the egg.
3. Arrange the avocado halves on the pan, hollow-side up. Break 1 egg into each half. Top each half with 1 tomato slice and ¼ cup of the Cottage cheese.
4. Slide the baking pan into Rack Position 1, select Convection Bake, set temperature to 425ºF (220ºC) and set time to 9 minutes.
5. When cooking is complete, remove the pan from the oven. Garnish with the fresh cilantro and serve.

54. Nutritious Egg Breakfast Muffins

Servings: 12
Cooking Time: 20 Minutes
Ingredients:
- 12 eggs
- 1/2 cup baby spinach, shredded
- 1 cup cheddar cheese, shredded
- 1/4 cup mushrooms, diced & sautéed
- 1/4 red bell pepper, diced
- 1/4 tsp garlic powder
- 1 cup ham, cooked and diced
- 3 tbsp onion, diced
- 1/2 tsp seasoned salt

Directions:
1. Fit the oven with the rack in position
2. Spray a 12-cup muffin tray with cooking spray and set aside.
3. In a large bowl, whisk eggs with garlic powder and salt.
4. Add remaining ingredients and stir well.
5. Pour egg mixture into the prepared muffin tray.
6. Set to bake at 350 F for 25 minutes. After 5 minutes place the muffin tray in the preheated oven.
7. Serve and enjoy.
Nutrition Info: Calories 122 Fat 8.5 g Carbohydrates 1.5 g Sugar 0.7 g Protein 9.9 g Cholesterol 180 mg

55. Rice, Shrimp, And Spinach Frittata

Servings: 4

Cooking Time: 16 Minutes
Ingredients:
- 4 eggs
- Pinch salt
- ½ cup cooked rice
- ½ cup chopped cooked shrimp
- ½ cup baby spinach
- ½ cup grated Monterey Jack cheese
- Nonstick cooking spray

Directions:
1. Spritz the baking pan with nonstick cooking spray.
2. Whisk the eggs and salt in a small bowl until frothy.
3. Place the cooked rice, shrimp, and baby spinach in the baking pan. Pour in the whisked eggs and scatter the cheese on top.
4. Slide the baking pan into Rack Position 1, select Convection Bake, set temperature to 320ºF (160ºC) and set time to 16 minutes.
5. When cooking is complete, the frittata should be golden and puffy.
6. Let the frittata cool for 5 minutes before slicing to serve.

56. Turkey, Leek, And Pepper Hamburger

Servings: 4
Cooking Time: 20 Minutes
Ingredients:
- 1 cup leftover turkey, cut into bite-sized chunks
- 1 leek, sliced
- 1 Serrano pepper, deveined and chopped
- 2 bell peppers, deveined and chopped
- 2 tablespoons Tabasco sauce
- ½ cup sour cream
- 1 heaping tablespoon fresh cilantro, chopped
- 1 teaspoon hot paprika
- ¾ teaspoon kosher salt
- ½ teaspoon ground black pepper
- 4 hamburger buns
- Cooking spray

Directions:
1. Spritz the baking pan with cooking spray.
2. Mix all the ingredients, except for the buns, in a large bowl. Toss to combine well.
3. Pour the mixture in the baking pan.
4. Slide the baking pan into Rack Position 1, select Convection Bake, set temperature to 385ºF (196ºC) and set time to 20 minutes.
5. When done, the turkey will be well browned and the leek will be tender.
6. Assemble the hamburger buns with the turkey mixture and serve immediately.

57. Air Fried French Toast

Servings: 4
Cooking Time: 6 Minutes

Ingredients:
- 2 slices of sourdough bread
- 3 eggs
- 1 tablespoon of margarine
- 1 tsp. of liquid vanilla
- 3 tsp.s of honey
- 2 tablespoons of Greek yogurt Berries

Directions:
1. Preheat the air fryer to 356°F.
2. Pour the vanilla in the eggs and whisk to mix. Spread the margarine on all sides of the bread and soak in the eggs to absorb.
3. Put the bread into the air fryer basket and cook for 3 minutes Turn the bread over and cook for another 3 minutes.
4. Transfer to a place, top with yogurt and berries with a sprinkle of honey.

Nutrition Info: Calories 99 Fat 8.2 g Carbohydrates 0.2 g Sugar 0.2 g Protein 6 g Cholesterol 18 mg

LUNCH RECIPES

58. Turkey-stuffed Peppers

Servings: 6
Cooking Time: 35 Minutes
Ingredients:
- 1 pound lean ground turkey
- 1 tablespoon olive oil
- 2 cloves garlic, minced
- 1/3 onion, minced
- 1 tablespoon cilantro (optional)
- 1 teaspoon garlic powder
- 1 teaspoon cumin powder
- 1/2 teaspoon salt
- Pepper to taste
- 3 large red bell peppers
- 1 cup chicken broth
- 1/4 cup tomato sauce
- 1-1/2 cups cooked brown rice
- 1/4 cup shredded cheddar
- 6 green onions

Directions:
1. Start by preheating toaster oven to 400°F.
2. Heat a skillet on medium heat.
3. Add olive oil to the skillet, then mix in onion and garlic.
4. Sauté for about 5 minutes, or until the onion starts to look opaque.
5. Add the turkey to the skillet and season with cumin, garlic powder, salt, and pepper.
6. Brown the meat until thoroughly cooked, then mix in chicken broth and tomato sauce.
7. Reduce heat and simmer for about 5 minutes, stirring occasionally.
8. Add the brown rice and continue stirring until it is evenly spread through the mix.
9. Cut the bell peppers lengthwise down the middle and remove all of the seeds.
10. Grease a pan or line it with parchment paper and lay all peppers in the pan with the outside facing down.
11. Spoon the meat mixture evenly into each pepper and use the back of the spoon to level.
12. Bake for 30 minutes.
13. Remove pan from oven and sprinkle cheddar over each pepper, then put it back in for another 3 minutes, or until the cheese is melted.
14. While the cheese melts, dice the green onions. Remove pan from oven and sprinkle onions over each pepper and serve.
Nutrition Info: Calories: 394, Sodium: 493 mg, Dietary Fiber: 4.1 g, Total Fat: 12.9 g, Total Carbs: 44.4 g, Protein: 27.7 g.

59. Lime And Mustard Marinated Chicken

Servings: 4
Cooking Time: 10 Minutes
Ingredients:
- 1/2 teaspoon stone-ground mustard
- 1/2 teaspoon minced fresh oregano
- 1/3 cup freshly squeezed lime juice
- 2 small-sized chicken breasts, skin-on
- 1 teaspoon kosher salt
- 1 teaspoon freshly cracked mixed peppercorns

Directions:
1. Preheat your Air Fryer to 345 degrees F.
2. Toss all of the above ingredients in a medium-sized mixing dish; allow it to marinate overnight.
3. Cook in the preheated Air Fryer for 26 minutes.
Nutrition Info: 255 Calories; 15g Fat; 7g Carbs; 33g Protein; 8g Sugars; 3g Fiber

60. Sweet Potato Rosti

Servings: 2
Cooking Time: 15 Minutes
Ingredients:
- ½ lb. sweet potatoes, peeled, grated and squeezed
- 1 tablespoon fresh parsley, chopped finely
- Salt and ground black pepper, as required
- 2 tablespoons sour cream

Directions:
1. In a large bowl, mix together the grated sweet potato, parsley, salt, and black pepper.
2. Press "Power Button" of Air Fry Oven and turn the dial to select the "Air Fry" mode.
3. Press the Time button and again turn the dial to set the cooking time to 15 minutes.
4. Now push the Temp button and rotate the dial to set the temperature at 355 degrees F.
5. Press "Start/Pause" button to start.
6. When the unit beeps to show that it is preheated, open the lid and lightly, grease the sheet pan.
7. Arrange the sweet potato mixture into the "Sheet Pan" and shape it into an even circle.
8. Insert the "Sheet Pan" in the oven.
9. Cut the potato rosti into wedges.
10. Top with the sour cream and serve immediately.
Nutrition Info: Calories: 160 Cal Total Fat: 2.7 g Saturated Fat: 1.6 g Cholesterol: 5 mg Sodium: 95 mg Total Carbs: 32.3 g Fiber: 4.7 g Sugar: 0.6 g Protein: 2.2 g

61. Garlic Chicken Potatoes

Servings: 4

Cooking Time: 30 Minutes
Ingredients:
- 2 lbs. red potatoes, quartered
- 3 tablespoons olive oil
- 1/2 teaspoon cumin seeds
- Salt and black pepper, to taste
- 4 garlic cloves, chopped
- 2 tablespoons brown sugar
- 1 lemon (1/2 juiced and 1/2 cut into wedges)
- Pinch of red pepper flakes
- 4 skinless, boneless chicken breasts
- 2 tablespoons cilantro, chopped

Directions:
1. Place the chicken, lemon, garlic, and potatoes in a baking pan.
2. Toss the spices, herbs, oil, and sugar in a bowl.
3. Add this mixture to the chicken and veggies then toss well to coat.
4. Press "Power Button" of Air Fry Oven and turn the dial to select the "Bake" mode.
5. Press the Time button and again turn the dial to set the cooking time to 30 minutes.
6. Now push the Temp button and rotate the dial to set the temperature at 400 degrees F.
7. Once preheated, place the baking pan inside and close its lid.
8. Serve warm.

Nutrition Info: Calories 545 Total Fat 36.4 g Saturated Fat 10.1 g Cholesterol 200 mg Sodium 272 mg Total Carbs 40.7 g Fiber 0.2 g Sugar 0.1 g Protein 42.5 g

62. Kalamta Mozarella Pita Melts

Servings: 2
Cooking Time: 5 Minutes
Ingredients:
- 2 (6-inch) whole wheat pitas
- 1 teaspoon extra-virgin olive oil
- 1 cup grated part-skim mozzarella cheese
- 1/4 small red onion
- 1/4 cup pitted Kalamata olives
- 2 tablespoons chopped fresh herbs such as parsley, basil, or oregano

Directions:
1. Start by preheating toaster oven to 425°F.
2. Brush the pita on both sides with oil and warm in the oven for one minute.
3. Dice onions and halve olives.
4. Sprinkle mozzarella over each pita and top with onion and olive.
5. Return to the oven for another 5 minutes or until the cheese is melted.
6. Sprinkle herbs over the pita and serve.

Nutrition Info: Calories: 387, Sodium: 828 mg, Dietary Fiber: 7.4 g, Total Fat: 16.2 g, Total Carbs: 42.0 g, Protein: 23.0 g.

63. Orange Chicken Rice

Servings: 4
Cooking Time: 55 Minutes
Ingredients:
- 3 tablespoons olive oil
- 1 medium onion, chopped
- 1 3/4 cups chicken broth
- 1 cup brown basmati rice
- Zest and juice of 2 oranges
- Salt to taste
- 4 (6-oz.) boneless, skinless chicken thighs
- Black pepper, to taste
- 2 tablespoons fresh mint, chopped
- 2 tablespoons pine nuts, toasted

Directions:
1. Spread the rice in a casserole dish and place the chicken on top.
2. Toss the rest of the Ingredients: in a bowl and liberally pour over the chicken.
3. Press "Power Button" of Air Fry Oven and turn the dial to select the "Bake" mode.
4. Press the Time button and again turn the dial to set the cooking time to 55 minutes.
5. Now push the Temp button and rotate the dial to set the temperature at 350 degrees F.
6. Once preheated, place the casserole dish inside and close its lid.
7. Serve warm.

Nutrition Info: Calories 231 Total Fat 20.1 g Saturated Fat 2.4 g Cholesterol 110 mg Sodium 941 mg Total Carbs 30.1 g Fiber 0.9 g Sugar 1.4 g Protein 14.6 g

64. Barbecue Air Fried Chicken

Servings: 10
Cooking Time: 26 Minutes
Ingredients:
- 1 teaspoon Liquid Smoke
- 2 cloves Fresh Garlic smashed
- 1/2 cup Apple Cider Vinegar
- 3 pounds Chuck Roast well-marbled with intramuscular fat
- 1 Tablespoon Kosher Salt
- 1 Tablespoon Freshly Ground Black Pepper
- 2 teaspoons Garlic Powder
- 1.5 cups Barbecue Sauce
- 1/4 cup Light Brown Sugar + more for sprinkling

- 2 Tablespoons Honey optional and in place of 2 TBL sugar

Directions:
1. Add meat to the Instant Pot Duo Crisp Air Fryer Basket, spreading out the meat.
2. Select the option Air Fry.
3. Close the Air Fryer lid and cook at 300 degrees F for 8 minutes. Pause the Air Fryer and flip meat over after 4 minutes.
4. Remove the lid and baste with more barbecue sauce and sprinkle with a little brown sugar.
5. Again Close the Air Fryer lid and set the temperature at 400°F for 9 minutes. Watch meat though the lid and flip it over after 5 minutes.

Nutrition Info: Calories 360, Total Fat 16g, Total Carbs 27g, Protein 27g

65. Duck Breast With Figs

Servings: 2
Cooking Time: 45 Minutes
Ingredients:
- 1 pound boneless duck breast
- 6 fresh figs, halved
- 1 tablespoon fresh thyme, chopped
- 2 cups fresh pomegranate juice
- 2 tablespoons lemon juice
- 3 tablespoons brown sugar
- 1 teaspoon olive oil
- Salt and black pepper, as required

Directions:
1. Preheat the Air fryer to 400 degree F and grease an Air fryer basket.
2. Put the pomegranate juice, lemon juice, and brown sugar in a medium saucepan over medium heat.
3. Bring to a boil and simmer on low heat for about 25 minutes.
4. Season the duck breasts generously with salt and black pepper.
5. Arrange the duck breasts into the Air fryer basket, skin side up and cook for about 14 minutes, flipping once in between.
6. Dish out the duck breasts onto a cutting board for about 10 minutes.
7. Meanwhile, put the figs, olive oil, salt, and black pepper in a bowl until well mixed.
8. Set the Air fryer to 400 degree F and arrange the figs into the Air fryer basket.
9. Cook for about 5 more minutes and dish out in a platter.
10. Put the duck breast with the roasted figs and drizzle with warm pomegranate juice mixture.
11. Garnish with fresh thyme and serve warm.

Nutrition Info: Calories: 699, Fat: 12.1g, Carbohydrates: 90g, Sugar: 74g, Protein: 519g, Sodium: 110mg

66. Glazed Lamb Chops

Servings: 4
Cooking Time: 15 Minutes
Ingredients:
- 1 tablespoon Dijon mustard
- ½ tablespoon fresh lime juice
- 1 teaspoon honey
- ½ teaspoon olive oil
- Salt and ground black pepper, as required
- 4 (4-ounce) lamb loin chops

Directions:
1. In a black pepper large bowl, mix together the mustard, lemon juice, oil, honey, salt, and black pepper.
2. Add the chops and coat with the mixture generously.
3. Place the chops onto the greased "Sheet Pan".
4. Press "Power Button" of Ninja Foodi Digital Air Fry Oven and turn the dial to select the "Air Bake" mode.
5. Press the Time button and again turn the dial to set the cooking time to 15 minutes.
6. Now push the Temp button and rotate the dial to set the temperature at 390 degrees F.
7. Press "Start/Pause" button to start.
8. When the unit beeps to show that it is preheated, open the lid.
9. Insert the "Sheet Pan" in oven.
10. Flip the chops once halfway through.
11. Serve hot.

Nutrition Info: Calories: 224 kcal Total Fat: 9.1 g Saturated Fat: 3.1 g Cholesterol: 102 mg Sodium: 169 mg Total Carbs: 1.7 g Fiber: 0.1 g Sugar: 1.5 g Protein: 32 g

67. Marinated Chicken Parmesan

Servings: 4
Cooking Time: 20 Minutes
Ingredients:
- 2 cups breadcrumbs
- 1 teaspoon dried oregano
- 1/2 teaspoon garlic powder
- 4 teaspoons paprika
- 1/2 teaspoon salt
- 1/2 teaspoon black pepper
- 2 egg whites
- 1/2 cup skim milk
- 1/2 cup flour
- 4 (6 oz.) chicken breast halves, lb.ed

- Cooking spray
- 1 jar marinara sauce
- 3/4 cup mozzarella cheese, shredded
- 2 tablespoons Parmesan, shredded

Directions:
1. Whisk the flour with all the spices in a bowl and beat the eggs in another.
2. Coat the pounded chicken with flour then dip in the egg whites.
3. Dredge the chicken breast through the crumbs well.
4. Spread marinara sauce in a baking dish and place the crusted chicken on it.
5. Drizzle cheese on top of the chicken.
6. Press "Power Button" of Air Fry Oven and turn the dial to select the "Bake" mode.
7. Press the Time button and again turn the dial to set the cooking time to 20 minutes.
8. Now push the Temp button and rotate the dial to set the temperature at 400 degrees F.
9. Once preheated, place the baking pan inside and close its lid.
10. Serve warm.

Nutrition Info: Calories 361 Total Fat 16.3 g Saturated Fat 4.9 g Cholesterol 114 mg Sodium 515 mg Total Carbs 19.3 g Fiber 0.1 g Sugar 18.2 g Protein 33.3 g

68. Kale And Pine Nuts

Servings: 4
Cooking Time: 12 Minutes
Ingredients:
- 10 cups kale; torn
- 1/3 cup pine nuts
- 2 tbsp. lemon zest; grated
- 1 tbsp. lemon juice
- 2 tbsp. olive oil
- Salt and black pepper to taste.

Directions:
1. In a pan that fits the air fryer, combine all the ingredients, toss, introduce the pan in the machine and cook at 380°F for 15 minutes
2. Divide between plates and serve as a side dish.

Nutrition Info: Calories: 121; Fat: 9g; Fiber: 2g; Carbs: 4g; Protein: 5g

69. Roasted Mini Peppers

Servings: 6
Cooking Time: 15 Minutes
Ingredients:
- 1 bag mini bell peppers
- Cooking spray
- Salt and pepper to taste

Directions:
1. Start by preheating toaster oven to 400°F.
2. Wash and dry the peppers, then place flat on a baking sheet.
3. Spray peppers with cooking spray and sprinkle with salt and pepper.
4. Roast for 15 minutes.

Nutrition Info: Calories: 19, Sodium: 2 mg, Dietary Fiber: 1.3 g, Total Fat: 0.3 g, Total Carbs: 3.6 g, Protein: 0.6 g.

70. Moroccan Pork Kebabs

Servings: 4
Cooking Time: 45 Minutes
Ingredients:
- 1/4 cup orange juice
- 1 tablespoon tomato paste
- 1 clove chopped garlic
- 1 tablespoon ground cumin
- 1/8 teaspoon ground cinnamon
- 4 tablespoons olive oil
- 1-1/2 teaspoons salt
- 3/4 teaspoon black pepper
- 1-1/2 pounds boneless pork loin
- 1 small eggplant
- 1 small red onion
- Pita bread (optional)
- 1/2 small cucumber
- 2 tablespoons chopped fresh mint
- Wooden skewers

Directions:
1. Start by placing wooden skewers in water to soak.
2. Cut pork loin and eggplant into 1- to 1-1/2-inch chunks.
3. Preheat toaster oven to 425°F.
4. Cut cucumber and onions into pieces and chop the mint.
5. In a large bowl, combine the orange juice, tomato paste, garlic, cumin, cinnamon, 2 tablespoons of oil, 1 teaspoon of salt, and 1/2 teaspoon of pepper.
6. Add the pork to this mixture and refrigerate for at least 30 minutes, but up to 8 hours.
7. Mix together vegetables, remaining oil, and salt and pepper.
8. Skewer the vegetables and bake for 20 minutes.
9. Add the pork to the skewers and bake for an additional 25 minutes.
10. Remove ingredients from skewers and sprinkle with mint; serve with flatbread if using.

Nutrition Info: Calories: 465, Sodium: 1061 mg, Dietary Fiber: 5.6 g, Total Fat: 20.8 g, Total Carbs: 21.9 g, Protein: 48.2 g.

71. Roasted Delicata Squash With Kale

Servings: 2
Cooking Time: 10 Minutes
Ingredients:
- 1 medium delicata squash
- 1 bunch kale
- 1 clove garlic
- 2 tablespoons olive oil
- Salt and pepper

Directions:
1. Start by preheating toaster oven to 425°F.
2. Clean squash and cut off each end. Cut in half and remove the seeds. Quarter the halves.
3. Toss the squash in 1 tablespoon of olive oil.
4. Place the squash on a greased baking sheet and roast for 25 minutes, turning halfway through.
5. Rinse kale and remove stems. Chop garlic.
6. Heat the leftover oil in a medium skillet and add kale and salt to taste.
7. Sauté the kale until it darkens, then mix in the garlic.
8. Cook for another minute then remove from heat and add 2 tablespoons of water.
9. Remove squash from oven and lay it on top of the garlic kale.
10. Top with salt and pepper to taste and serve.
Nutrition Info: Calories: 159, Sodium: 28 mg, Dietary Fiber: 1.8 g, Total Fat: 14.2 g, Total Carbs: 8.2 g, Protein: 2.6 g.

72. Spicy Avocado Cauliflower Toast

Servings: 2
Cooking Time: 15 Minutes
Ingredients:
- 1/2 large head of cauliflower, leaves removed
- 3 1/4 teaspoons olive oil
- 1 small jalapeño
- 1 tablespoon chopped cilantro leaves
- 2 slices whole grain bread
- 1 medium avocado
- Salt and pepper
- 5 radishes
- 1 green onion
- 2 teaspoons hot sauce
- 1 lime

Directions:
1. Start by preheating toaster oven to 450°F.
2. Cut cauliflower into thick pieces, about 3/4-inches-thick, and slice jalapeño into thin slices.
3. Place cauliflower and jalapeño in a bowl and mix together with 2 teaspoons olive oil.
4. Add salt and pepper to taste and mix for another minute.

5. Coat a pan with another teaspoon of olive oil, then lay the cauliflower mixture flat across the pan.
6. Cook for 20 minutes, flipping in the last 5 minutes.
7. Reduce heat to toast.
8. Sprinkle cilantro over the mix while it is still warm, and set aside.
9. Brush bread with remaining oil and toast until golden brown, about 5 minutes.
10. Dice onion and radish.
11. Mash avocado in a bowl, then spread on toast and sprinkle salt and pepper to taste.
12. Put cauliflower mix on toast and cover with onion and radish. Drizzle with hot sauce and serve with a lime wedge.
Nutrition Info: Calories: 359, Sodium: 308 mg, Dietary Fiber: 11.1 g, Total Fat: 28.3 g, Total Carbs: 26.4 g, Protein: 6.6 g.

73. Philly Cheesesteak Egg Rolls

Servings: 4-5
Cooking Time: 20 Minutes
Ingredients:
- 1 egg
- 1 tablespoon milk
- 2 tablespoons olive oil
- 1 small red onion
- 1 small red bell pepper
- 1 small green bell pepper
- 1 pound thinly slice roast beef
- 8 ounces shredded pepper jack cheese
- 8 ounces shredded provolone cheese
- 8-10 egg roll skins
- Salt and pepper

Directions:
1. Start by preheating toaster oven to 425°F.
2. Mix together egg and milk in a shallow bowl and set aside for later use.
3. Chop onions and bell peppers into small pieces.
4. Heat the oil in a medium sauce pan and add the onions and peppers.
5. Cook onions and peppers for 2–3 minutes until softened.
6. Add roast beef to the pan and sauté for another 5 minutes.
7. Add salt and pepper to taste.
8. Add cheese and mix together until melted.
9. Remove from heat and drain liquid from pan.
10. Roll the egg roll skins flat.
11. Add equal parts of the mix to each egg roll and roll them up per the instructions on the package.
12. Brush each egg roll with the egg mixture.
13. Line a pan with parchment paper and lay egg rolls seam-side down with a gap between each roll.

14. Bake for 20–25 minutes, depending on your preference of egg roll crispness.

Nutrition Info: Calories: 769, Sodium: 1114 mg, Dietary Fiber: 2.1 g, Total Fat: 39.9 g, Total Carbs: 41.4 g, Protein: 58.4 g.

74. Spicy Egg And Ground Turkey Bake

Servings: 6
Cooking Time: 10 Minutes
Ingredients:
- 1½ pounds ground turkey
- 6 whole eggs, well beaten
- 1/3 teaspoon smoked paprika
- 2 egg whites, beaten
- Tabasco sauce, for drizzling
- 2 tablespoons sesame oil
- 2 leeks, chopped
- 3 cloves garlic, finely minced
- 1 teaspoon ground black pepper
- 1/2 teaspoon sea salt

Directions:
1. Warm the oil in a pan over moderate heat; then, sweat the leeks and garlic until tender; stir periodically.
2. Next, grease 6 oven safe ramekins with pan spray. Divide the sautéed mixture among six ramekins.
3. In a bowl, beat the eggs and egg whites using a wire whisk. Stir in the smoked paprika, salt and black pepper; whisk until everything is thoroughly combined. Divide the egg mixture among the ramekins.
4. Air-fry approximately 22 minutes at 345 degrees F. Drizzle Tabasco sauce over each portion and serve.

Nutrition Info: 298 Calories; 16g Fat; 4g Carbs; 16g Protein; 9g Sugars; 7g Fiber

75. Deviled Chicken

Servings: 8
Cooking Time: 40 Minutes
Ingredients:
- 2 tablespoons butter
- 2 cloves garlic, chopped
- 1 cup Dijon mustard
- 1/2 teaspoon cayenne pepper
- 1 1/2 cups panko breadcrumbs
- 3/4 cup Parmesan, freshly grated
- 1/4 cup chives, chopped
- 2 teaspoons paprika
- 8 small bone-in chicken thighs, skin removed

Directions:
1. Toss the chicken thighs with crumbs, cheese, chives, butter, and spices in a bowl and mix well to coat.
2. Transfer the chicken along with its spice mix to a baking pan.
3. Press "Power Button" of Air Fry Oven and turn the dial to select the "Air Fry" mode.
4. Press the Time button and again turn the dial to set the cooking time to 40 minutes.
5. Now push the Temp button and rotate the dial to set the temperature at 350 degrees F.
6. Once preheated, place the baking pan inside and close its lid.
7. Serve warm.

Nutrition Info: Calories 380 Total Fat 20 g Saturated Fat 5 g Cholesterol 151 mg Sodium 686 mg Total Carbs 33 g Fiber 1 g Sugar 1.2 g Protein 21 g

76. Chicken Legs With Dilled Brussels Sprouts

Servings: 2
Cooking Time: 10 Minutes
Ingredients:
- 2 chicken legs
- 1/2 teaspoon paprika
- 1/2 teaspoon kosher salt
- 1/2 teaspoon black pepper
- 1/2 pound Brussels sprouts
- 1 teaspoon dill, fresh or dried

Directions:
1. Start by preheating your Air Fryer to 370 degrees F.
2. Now, season your chicken with paprika, salt, and pepper. Transfer the chicken legs to the cooking basket. Cook for 10 minutes.
3. Flip the chicken legs and cook an additional 10 minutes. Reserve.
4. Add the Brussels sprouts to the cooking basket; sprinkle with dill. Cook at 380 degrees F for 15 minutes, shaking the basket halfway through.
5. Serve with the reserved chicken legs.

Nutrition Info: 365 Calories; 21g Fat; 3g Carbs; 36g Protein; 2g Sugars; 3g Fiber

77. Lamb Gyro

Servings: 4
Cooking Time: 25 Minutes
Ingredients:
- 1 pound ground lamb
- ¼ red onion, minced
- ¼ cup mint, minced
- ¼ cup parsley, minced
- 2 cloves garlic, minced

- ½ teaspoon salt
- ⅛ teaspoon rosemary
- ½ teaspoon black pepper
- 4 slices pita bread
- ¾ cup hummus
- 1 cup romaine lettuce, shredded
- ½ onion sliced
- 1 Roma tomato, diced
- ½ cucumber, skinned and thinly sliced
- 12 mint leaves, minced
- Tzatziki sauce, to taste

Directions:
1. Mix ground lamb, red onion, mint, parsley, garlic, salt, rosemary, and black pepper until fully incorporated.
2. Select the Broil function on the COSORI Air Fryer Toaster Oven, set time to 25 minutes and temperature to 450°F, then press Start/Cancel to preheat.
3. Line the food tray with parchment paper and place ground lamb on top, shaping it into a patty 1-inch-thick and 6 inches in diameter.
4. Insert the food tray at top position in the preheated air fryer toaster oven, then press Start/Cancel.
5. Remove when done and cut into thin slices.
6. Assemble each gyro starting with pita bread, then hummus, lamb meat, lettuce, onion, tomato, cucumber, and mint leaves, then drizzle with tzatziki.
7. Serve immediately.

Nutrition Info: Calories: 409 kcal Total Fat: 14.6 g Saturated Fat: 0 g Cholesterol: 0 mg Sodium: 0 mg Total Carbs: 29.9 g Fiber: 0 g Sugar: 0 g Protein: 39.4 g

78. Tomato Avocado Melt

Servings: 2
Cooking Time: 4 Minutes
Ingredients:
- 4 slices of bread
- 1-2 tablespoons mayonnaise
- Cayenne pepper
- 1 small Roma tomato
- 1/2 avocado
- 8 slices of cheese of your choice

Directions:
1. Start by slicing avocado and tomato and set aside.
2. Spread mayonnaise on the bread.
3. Sprinkle cayenne pepper over the mayo to taste.
4. Layer tomato and avocado on top of cayenne pepper.
5. Top with cheese and put on greased baking sheet.

6. Broil on high for 2–4 minutes, until the cheese is melted and bread is toasted.
Nutrition Info: Calories: 635, Sodium: 874 mg, Dietary Fiber: 4.1 g, Total Fat: 50.1 g, Total Carbs: 17.4 g, Protein: 30.5 g.

79. Coriander Artichokes(3)

Servings: 4
Cooking Time: 12 Minutes
Ingredients:
- 12 oz. artichoke hearts
- 1 tbsp. lemon juice
- 1 tsp. coriander, ground
- ½ tsp. cumin seeds
- ½ tsp. olive oil
- Salt and black pepper to taste.

Directions:
1. In a pan that fits your air fryer, mix all the ingredients, toss, introduce the pan in the fryer and cook at 370°F for 15 minutes
2. Divide the mix between plates and serve as a side dish.
Nutrition Info: Calories: 200; Fat: 7g; Fiber: 2g; Carbs: 5g; Protein: 8g

80. Chicken Breast With Rosemary

Servings: 4
Cooking Time: 60 Minutes
Ingredients:
- 4 bone-in chicken breast halves
- 3 tablespoons softened butter
- 1/2 teaspoon salt
- 1/4 teaspoon pepper
- 1 tablespoon rosemary
- 1 tablespoon extra-virgin olive oil

Directions:
1. Start by preheating toaster oven to 400°F.
2. Mix butter, salt, pepper, and rosemary in a bowl.
3. Coat chicken with the butter mixture and place in a shallow pan.
4. Drizzle oil over chicken and roast for 25 minutes.
5. Flip chicken and roast for another 20 minutes.
6. Flip chicken one more time and roast for a final 15 minutes.
Nutrition Info: Calories: 392, Sodium: 551 mg, Dietary Fiber: 0 g, Total Fat: 18.4 g, Total Carbs: 0.6 g, Protein: 55.4 g.

81. Beef Steaks With Beans

Servings: 4
Cooking Time: 10 Minutes
Ingredients:

- 4 beef steaks, trim the fat and cut into strips
- 1 cup green onions, chopped
- 2 cloves garlic, minced
- 1 red bell pepper, seeded and thinly sliced
- 1 can tomatoes, crushed
- 1 can cannellini beans
- 3/4 cup beef broth
- 1/4 teaspoon dried basil
- 1/2 teaspoon cayenne pepper
- 1/2 teaspoon sea salt
- 1/4 teaspoon ground black pepper, or to taste

Directions:
1. Preparing the ingredients. Add the steaks, green onions and garlic to the instant crisp air fryer basket.
2. Air frying. Close air fryer lid. Cook at 390 degrees f for 10 minutes, working in batches.
3. Stir in the remaining ingredients and cook for an additional 5 minutes.

Nutrition Info: Calories 284 Total fat 7.9 g Saturated fat 1.4 g Cholesterol 36 mg Sodium 704 mg Total carbs 46 g Fiber 3.6 g Sugar 5.5 g Protein 17.9 g

82. Sweet Potato And Parsnip Spiralized Latkes

Servings: 12
Cooking Time: 20 Minutes
Ingredients:
- 1 medium sweet potato
- 1 large parsnip
- 4 cups water
- 1 egg + 1 egg white
- 2 scallions
- 1/2 teaspoon garlic powder
- 1/2 teaspoon sea salt
- 1/2 teaspoon ground pepper

Directions:
1. Start by spiralizing the sweet potato and parsnip and chopping the scallions, reserving only the green parts.
2. Preheat toaster oven to 425°F.
3. Bring 4 cups of water to a boil. Place all of your noodles in a colander and pour the boiling water over the top, draining well.
4. Let the noodles cool, then grab handfuls and place them in a paper towel; squeeze to remove as much liquid as possible.
5. In a large bowl, beat egg and egg white together. Add noodles, scallions, garlic powder, salt, and pepper, mix well.
6. Prepare a baking sheet; scoop out 1/4 cup of mixture at a time and place on sheet.
7. Slightly press down each scoop with your hands, then bake for 20 minutes, flipping halfway through.

Nutrition Info: Calories: 24, Sodium: 91 mg, Dietary Fiber: 1.0 g, Total Fat: 0.4 g, Total Carbs: 4.3 g, Protein: 0.9 g.

83. Crispy Breaded Pork Chop

Servings: 6
Cooking Time: 12 Minutes
Ingredients:
- olive oil spray
- 6 3/4-inch thick center-cut boneless pork chops, fat trimmed (5 oz each)
- kosher salt
- 1 large egg, beaten
- 1/2 cup panko crumbs, check labels for GF
- 1/3 cup crushed cornflakes crumbs
- 2 tbsp grated parmesan cheese
- 1 1/4 tsp sweet paprika
- 1/2 tsp garlic powder
- 1/2 tsp onion powder
- 1/4 tsp chili powder
- 1/8 tsp black pepper

Directions:
1. Preheat the Instant Pot Duo Crisp Air Fryer for 12 minutes at 400°F.
2. On both sides, season pork chops with half teaspoon kosher salt.
3. Then combine cornflake crumbs, panko, parmesan cheese, 3/4 tsp kosher salt, garlic powder, paprika, onion powder, chili powder, and black pepper in a large bowl.
4. Place the egg beat in another bowl. Dip the pork in the egg & then crumb mixture.
5. When the air fryer is ready, place 3 of the chops into the Instant Pot Duo Crisp Air Fryer Basket and spritz the top with oil.
6. Close the Air Fryer lid and cook for 12 minutes turning halfway, spritzing both sides with oil.
7. Set aside and repeat with the remaining.

Nutrition Info: Calories 281, Total Fat 13g, Total Carbs 8g, Protein 33g

84. Portobello Pesto Burgers

Servings: 4
Cooking Time: 26 Minutes
Ingredients:
- 4 portobello mushrooms
- 1/4 cup sundried tomato pesto
- 4 whole-grain hamburger buns
- 1 large ripe tomato
- 1 log fresh goat cheese
- 8 large fresh basil leaves

Directions:
1. Start by preheating toaster oven to 425°F.

2. Place mushrooms on a pan, round sides facing up.
3. Bake for 14 minutes.
4. Pull out tray, flip the mushrooms and spread 1 tablespoon of pesto on each piece.
5. Return to oven and bake for another 10 minutes.
6. Remove the mushrooms and toast the buns for 2 minutes.
7. Remove the buns and build the burger by placing tomatoes, mushroom, 2 slices of cheese, and a sprinkle of basil, then topping with the top bun.
Nutrition Info: Calories: 297, Sodium: 346 mg, Dietary Fiber: 1.8 g, Total Fat: 18.1 g, Total Carbs: 19.7 g, Protein: 14.4 g.

85. Vegetarian Philly Sandwich

Servings: 2
Cooking Time: 20 Minutes
Ingredients:
- 2 tablespoons olive oil
- 8 ounces sliced portabello mushrooms
- 1 vidalia onion, thinly sliced
- 1 green bell pepper, thinly sliced
- 1 red bell pepper, thinly sliced
- Salt and pepper
- 4 slices 2% provolone cheese
- 4 rolls

Directions:
1. Preheat toaster oven to 475°F.
2. Heat the oil in a medium sauce pan over medium heat.
3. Sauté mushrooms about 5 minutes, then add the onions and peppers and sauté another 10 minutes.
4. Slice rolls lengthwise and divide the vegetables into each roll.
5. Add the cheese and toast until the rolls start to brown and the cheese melts.
Nutrition Info: Calories: 645, Sodium: 916 mg, Dietary Fiber: 7.2 g, Total Fat: 33.3 g, Total Carbs: 61.8 g, Protein: 27.1 g.

86. Fried Whole Chicken

Servings: 4
Cooking Time: 70 Minutes
Ingredients:
- 1 Whole chicken
- 2 Tbsp or spray of oil of choice
- 1 tsp garlic powder
- 1 tsp onion powder
- 1 tsp paprika
- 1 tsp Italian seasoning
- 2 Tbsp Montreal Steak Seasoning (or salt and pepper to taste)

- 1.5 cup chicken broth

Directions:
1. Truss and wash the chicken.
2. Mix the seasoning and rub a little amount on the chicken.
3. Pour the broth inside the Instant Pot Duo Crisp Air Fryer.
4. Place the chicken in the air fryer basket.
5. Select the option Air Fry and Close the Air Fryer lid and cook for 25 minutes.
6. Spray or rub the top of the chicken with oil and rub it with half of the seasoning.
7. Close the air fryer lid and air fry again at 400°F for 10 minutes.
8. Flip the chicken, spray it with oil, and rub with the remaining seasoning.
9. Again air fry it for another ten minutes.
10. Allow the chicken to rest for 10 minutes.
Nutrition Info: Calories 436, Total Fat 28g, Total Carbs 4g, Protein 42g

87. Cheese-stuffed Meatballs

Servings: 4
Cooking Time: 10 Minutes
Ingredients:
- ⅓ cup soft bread crumbs
- 3 tablespoons milk
- 1 tablespoon ketchup
- 1 egg
- ½ teaspoon dried marjoram
- Pinch salt
- Freshly ground black pepper
- 1-pound 95 percent lean ground beef
- 20 ½-inch cubes of cheese
- Olive oil for misting

Directions:
1. Preparing the ingredients. In a large bowl, combine the bread crumbs, milk, ketchup, egg, marjoram, salt, and pepper, and mix well. Add the ground beef and mix gently but thoroughly with your hands. Form the mixture into 20 meatballs. Shape each meatball around a cheese cube. Mist the meatballs with olive oil and put into the instant crisp air fryer basket.
2. Air frying. Close air fryer lid. Bake for 10 to 13 minutes or until the meatballs register 165°f on a meat thermometer.
Nutrition Info: Calories: 393; Fat: 17g; Protein:50g; Fiber:0g

88. Green Bean Casserole(2)

Servings: 4
Cooking Time: 12 Minutes

Ingredients:

- 1 lb. fresh green beans, edges trimmed
- ½ oz. pork rinds, finely ground
- 1 oz. full-fat cream cheese
- ½ cup heavy whipping cream.
- ¼ cup diced yellow onion
- ½ cup chopped white mushrooms
- ½ cup chicken broth
- 4 tbsp. unsalted butter.
- ¼ tsp. xanthan gum

Directions:

1. In a medium skillet over medium heat, melt the butter. Sauté the onion and mushrooms until they become soft and fragrant, about 3–5 minutes.
2. Add the heavy whipping cream, cream cheese and broth to the pan. Whisk until smooth. Bring to a boil and then reduce to a simmer. Sprinkle the xanthan gum into the pan and remove from heat
3. Chop the green beans into 2-inch pieces and place into a 4-cup round baking dish. Pour the sauce mixture over them and stir until coated. Top the dish with ground pork rinds. Place into the air fryer basket
4. Adjust the temperature to 320 Degrees F and set the timer for 15 minutes. Top will be golden and green beans fork tender when fully cooked. Serve warm.

Nutrition Info: Calories: 267; Protein: 6g; Fiber: 2g; Fat: 24g; Carbs: 7g

89. Turmeric Mushroom(3)

Servings: 4
Cooking Time: 12 Minutes
Ingredients:

- 1 lb. brown mushrooms
- 4 garlic cloves; minced
- ¼ tsp. cinnamon powder
- 1 tsp. olive oil
- ½ tsp. turmeric powder
- Salt and black pepper to taste.

Directions:

1. In a bowl, combine all the ingredients and toss.
2. Put the mushrooms in your air fryer's basket and cook at 370°F for 15 minutes
3. Divide the mix between plates and serve as a side dish.

Nutrition Info: Calories: 208; Fat: 7g; Fiber: 3g; Carbs: 5g; Protein: 7g

90. Bbq Chicken Breasts

Servings: 4
Cooking Time: 15 Minutes
Ingredients:

- 4 boneless skinless chicken breast about 6 oz each
- 1-2 Tbsp bbq seasoning

Directions:

1. Cover both sides of chicken breast with the BBQ seasoning. Cover and marinate the in the refrigerator for 45 minutes.
2. Choose the Air Fry option and set the temperature to 400°F. Push start and let it preheat for 5 minutes.
3. Upon preheating, place the chicken breast in the Instant Pot Duo Crisp Air Fryer basket, making sure they do not overlap. Spray with oil.
4. Cook for 13-14 minutes
5. flipping halfway.
6. Remove chicken when the chicken reaches an internal temperature of 160°F. Place on a plate and allow to rest for 5 minutes before slicing.

Nutrition Info: Calories 131, Total Fat 3g, Total Carbs 2g, Protein 24g

91. Parmesan-crusted Pork Loin

Servings: 4
Cooking Time: 20 Minutes
Ingredients:

- 1 pound pork loin
- 1 teaspoon salt
- 1/2 tablespoon garlic powder
- 1/2 tablespoon onion powder
- 2 tablespoons parmesan cheese
- 1 tablespoon olive oil

Directions:

1. Start by preheating toaster oven to 475°F.
2. Place pan in the oven and let it heat while the oven preheats.
3. Mix all ingredients in a shallow dish and roll the pork loin until it is fully coated.
4. Remove pan and sear the pork in the pan on each side.
5. Once seared, bake pork in the pan for 20 minutes.

Nutrition Info: Calories: 334, Sodium: 718 mg, Dietary Fiber: 0 g, Total Fat: 20.8 g, Total Carbs: 1.7 g, Protein: 33.5 g.

92. Sweet Potato And Eggplant Mix

Servings: 4
Cooking Time: 20 Minutes
Ingredients:

- 2 sweet potatoes, peeled and cut into medium wedges
- 2 eggplants, roughly cubed
- 1 tablespoon avocado oil

- Juice of 1 lemon
- 4 garlic cloves, minced
- 1 teaspoon nutmeg, ground
- Salt and black pepper to the taste
- 1 tablespoon rosemary, chopped

Directions:
1. In your air fryer, combine the potatoes with the eggplants and the other Ingredients:, toss and cook at 370 degrees F for 20 minutes.
2. Divide the mix between plates and serve as a side dish.

Nutrition Info: Calories 182, fat 6, fiber 3, carbs 11, protein 5

93. Herbed Radish Sauté(3)

Servings: 4
Cooking Time: 12 Minutes
Ingredients:
- 2 bunches red radishes; halved
- 2 tbsp. parsley; chopped.
- 2 tbsp. balsamic vinegar
- 1 tbsp. olive oil
- Salt and black pepper to taste.

Directions:
1. Take a bowl and mix the radishes with the remaining ingredients except the parsley, toss and put them in your air fryer's basket.
2. Cook at 400°F for 15 minutes, divide between plates, sprinkle the parsley on top and serve as a side dish

Nutrition Info: Calories: 180; Fat: 4g; Fiber: 2g; Carbs: 3g; Protein: 5g

94. Zucchini And Cauliflower Stew

Servings: 4
Cooking Time: 12 Minutes
Ingredients:
- 1 cauliflower head, florets separated
- 1 ½ cups zucchinis; sliced
- 1 handful parsley leaves; chopped.
- ½ cup tomato puree
- 2 green onions; chopped.
- 1 tbsp. balsamic vinegar
- 1 tbsp. olive oil
- Salt and black pepper to taste.

Directions:
1. In a pan that fits your air fryer, mix the zucchinis with the rest of the ingredients except the parsley, toss, introduce the pan in the air fryer and cook at 380°F for 20 minutes
2. Divide into bowls and serve for lunch with parsley sprinkled on top.

Nutrition Info: Calories: 193; Fat: 5g; Fiber: 2g; Carbs: 4g; Protein: 7g

95. Turkey And Almonds

Servings: 2
Cooking Time: 10 Minutes
Ingredients:
- 1 big turkey breast, skinless; boneless and halved
- 2 shallots; chopped
- 1/3 cup almonds; chopped
- 1 tbsp. sweet paprika
- 2 tbsp. olive oil
- Salt and black pepper to taste.

Directions:
1. In a pan that fits the air fryer, combine the turkey with all the other ingredients, toss.
2. Put the pan in the machine and cook at 370°F for 25 minutes
3. Divide everything between plates and serve.

Nutrition Info: Calories: 274; Fat: 12g; Fiber: 3g; Carbs: 5g; Protein: 14g

96. Baked Shrimp Scampi

Servings: 4
Cooking Time: 10 Minutes
Ingredients:
- 1 lb large shrimp
- 8 tbsp butter
- 1 tbsp minced garlic (use 2 for extra garlic flavor)
- 1/4 cup white wine or cooking sherry
- 1/2 tsp salt
- 1/4 tsp cayenne pepper
- 1/4 tsp paprika
- 1/2 tsp onion powder
- 3/4 cup bread crumbs

Directions:
1. Take a bowl and mix the bread crumbs with dry seasonings.
2. On the stovetop (or in the Instant Pot on saute), melt the butter with the garlic and the white wine.
3. Remove from heat and add the shrimp and the bread crumb mix.
4. Transfer the mix to a casserole dish.
5. Choose the Bake operation and add food to the Instant Pot Duo Crisp Air Fryer. Close the lid and Bake at 350°F for 10 minutes or until they are browned.
6. Serve and enjoy.

Nutrition Info: Calories 422, Total Fat 26g, Total Carbs 18g, Protein 29 g

97. Sweet Potato Chips

Servings: 2
Cooking Time: 40 Minutes
Ingredients:
- 2 sweet potatoes
- Salt and pepper to taste
- Olive oil
- Cinnamon

Directions:
1. Start by preheating toaster oven to 400°F.
2. Cut off each end of potato and discard.
3. Cut potatoes into 1/2-inch slices.
4. Brush a pan with olive oil and lay potato slices flat on the pan.
5. Bake for 20 minutes, then flip and bake for another 20.

Nutrition Info: Calories: 139, Sodium: 29 mg, Dietary Fiber: 8.2 g, Total Fat: 0.5 g, Total Carbs: 34.1 g, Protein: 1.9 g.

98. Chicken Caprese Sandwich

Servings: 2
Cooking Time: 3 Minutes
Ingredients:
- 2 leftover chicken breasts, or pre-cooked breaded chicken
- 1 large ripe tomato
- 4 ounces mozzarella cheese slices
- 4 slices of whole grain bread
- 1/4 cup olive oil
- 1/3 cup fresh basil leaves
- Salt and pepper to taste

Directions:
1. Start by slicing tomatoes into thin slices.
2. Layer tomatoes then cheese over two slices of bread and place on a greased baking sheet.
3. Toast in the toaster oven for about 2 minutes or until the cheese is melted.
4. Heat chicken while the cheese melts.
5. Remove from oven, sprinkle with basil, and add chicken.
6. Drizzle with oil and add salt and pepper.
7. Top with other slice of bread and serve.

Nutrition Info: Calories: 808, Sodium: 847 mg, Dietary Fiber: 5.2 g, Total Fat: 43.6 g, Total Carbs: 30.7 g, Protein: 78.4 g.

99. Mushroom Meatloaf

Servings: 4
Cooking Time: 25 Minutes
Ingredients:
- 14-ounce lean ground beef
- 1 chorizo sausage, chopped finely
- 1 small onion, chopped
- 1 garlic clove, minced
- 2 tablespoons fresh cilantro, chopped
- 3 tablespoons breadcrumbs
- 1 egg
- Salt and freshly ground black pepper, to taste
- 2 tablespoons fresh mushrooms, sliced thinly
- 3 tablespoons olive oil

Directions:
1. Preparing the ingredients. Preheat the instant crisp air fryer to 390 degrees f.
2. In a large bowl, add all ingredients except mushrooms and mix till well combined.
3. In a baking pan, place the beef mixture.
4. With the back of spatula, smooth the surface.
5. Top with mushroom slices and gently, press into the meatloaf.
6. Drizzle with oil evenly.
7. Air frying. Arrange the pan in the instant crisp air fryer basket, close air fryer lid and cook for about 25 minutes.
8. Cut the meatloaf in desires size wedges and serve.

Nutrition Info: Calories 284 Total fat 7.9 g Saturated fat 1.4 g Cholesterol 36 mg Sodium 704 mg Total carbs 46 g Fiber 3.6 g Sugar 5.5 g Protein 17.9 g

100. Turkey Meatloaf

Servings: 4
Cooking Time: 20 Minutes
Ingredients:
- 1 pound ground turkey
- 1 cup kale leaves, trimmed and finely chopped
- 1 cup onion, chopped
- ½ cup fresh breadcrumbs
- 1 cup Monterey Jack cheese, grated
- 2 garlic cloves, minced
- ¼ cup salsa verde
- 1 teaspoon red chili powder
- ½ teaspoon ground cumin
- ½ teaspoon dried oregano, crushed
- Salt and ground black pepper, as required

Directions:
1. Preheat the Air fryer to 400 degree F and grease an Air fryer basket.
2. Mix all the ingredients in a bowl and divide the turkey mixture into 4 equal-sized portions.
3. Shape each into a mini loaf and arrange the loaves into the Air fryer basket.
4. Cook for about 20 minutes and dish out to serve warm.

Nutrition Info: Calories: 435, Fat: 23.1g, Carbohydrates: 18.1g, Sugar: 3.6g, Protein: 42.2g, Sodium: 641mg

101.Basic Roasted Tofu

Servings: 4
Cooking Time: 45 Minutes
Ingredients:
- 1 or more (16-ounce) containers extra-firm tofu
- 1 tablespoon sesame oil
- 1 tablespoon soy sauce
- 1 tablespoon rice vinegar
- 1 tablespoon water

Directions:
1. Start by drying the tofu: first pat dry with paper towels, then lay on another set of paper towels or a dish towel.
2. Put a plate on top of the tofu then put something heavy on the plate (like a large can of vegetables). Leave it there for at least 20 minutes.
3. While tofu is being pressed, whip up marinade by combining oil, soy sauce, vinegar, and water in a bowl and set aside.
4. Cut the tofu into squares or sticks. Place the tofu in the marinade for at least 30 minutes.
5. Preheat toaster oven to 350°F. Line a pan with parchment paper and add as many pieces of tofu as you can, giving each piece adequate space.
6. Bake 20–45 minutes; tofu is done when the outside edges look golden brown. Time will vary depending on tofu size and shape.
Nutrition Info: Calories: 114, Sodium: 239 mg, Dietary Fiber: 1.1 g, Total Fat: 8.1 g, Total Carbs: 2.2 g, Protein: 9.5 g.

102.Easy Prosciutto Grilled Cheese

Servings: 1
Cooking Time: 5 Minutes
Ingredients:
- 2 slices muenster cheese
- 2 slices white bread
- Four thinly-shaved pieces of prosciutto
- 1 tablespoon sweet and spicy pickles

Directions:
1. Set toaster oven to the Toast setting.
2. Place one slice of cheese on each piece of bread.
3. Put prosciutto on one slice and pickles on the other.
4. Transfer to a baking sheet and toast for 4 minutes or until the cheese is melted.
5. Combine the sides, cut, and serve.
Nutrition Info: Calories: 460, Sodium: 2180 mg, Dietary Fiber: 0 g, Total Fat: 25.2 g, Total Carbs: 11.9 g, Protein: 44.2 g.

103.Lobster Tails

Servings: 2
Cooking Time: 8 Minutes
Ingredients:
- 2 6oz lobster tails
- 1 tsp salt
- 1 tsp chopped chives
- 2 Tbsp unsalted butter melted
- 1 Tbsp minced garlic
- 1 tsp lemon juice

Directions:
1. Combine butter, garlic, salt, chives, and lemon juice to prepare butter mixture.
2. Butterfly lobster tails by cutting through shell followed by removing the meat and resting it on top of the shell.
3. Place them on the tray in the Instant Pot Duo Crisp Air Fryer basket and spread butter over the top of lobster meat. Close the Air Fryer lid, select the Air Fry option and cook on 380°F for 4 minutes.
4. Open the Air Fryer lid and spread more butter on top, cook for extra 2-4 minutes until done.
Nutrition Info: Calories 120, Total Fat 12g, Total Carbs 2g, Protein 1g

104.Buttered Duck Breasts

Servings: 4
Cooking Time: 22 Minutes
Ingredients:
- 2: 12-ouncesduck breasts
- 3 tablespoons unsalted butter, melted
- Salt and ground black pepper, as required
- ½ teaspoon dried thyme, crushed
- ¼ teaspoon star anise powder

Directions:
1. Preheat the Air fryer to 390 degree F and grease an Air fryer basket.
2. Season the duck breasts generously with salt and black pepper.
3. Arrange the duck breasts into the prepared Air fryer basket and cook for about 10 minutes.
4. Dish out the duck breasts and drizzle with melted butter.
5. Season with thyme and star anise powder and place the duck breasts again into the Air fryer basket.
6. Cook for about 12 more minutes and dish out to serve warm.
Nutrition Info: Calories: 296, Fat: 15.5g, Carbohydrates: 0.1g, Sugar: 0g, Protein: 37.5g, Sodium: 100mg

105.Turkey And Broccoli Stew

Servings: 4

Cooking Time: 12 Minutes
Ingredients:
- 1 broccoli head, florets separated
- 1 turkey breast, skinless; boneless and cubed
- 1 cup tomato sauce
- 1 tbsp. parsley; chopped.
- 1 tbsp. olive oil
- Salt and black pepper to taste.

Directions:
1. In a baking dish that fits your air fryer, mix the turkey with the rest of the ingredients except the parsley, toss, introduce the dish in the fryer, bake at 380°F for 25 minutes
2. Divide into bowls, sprinkle the parsley on top and serve.

Nutrition Info: Calories: 250; Fat: 11g; Fiber: 2g; Carbs: 6g; Protein: 12g

106.Persimmon Toast With Sour Cream & Cinnamon

Servings: 1
Cooking Time: 5 Minutes
Ingredients:
- 1 slice of wheat bread
- 1/2 persimmon
- Sour cream to taste
- Sugar to taste
- Cinnamon to taste

Directions:
1. Spread a thin layer of sour cream across the bread.
2. Slice the persimmon into 1/4 inch pieces and lay them across the bread.
3. Sprinkle cinnamon and sugar over persimmon.
4. Toast in toaster oven until bread and persimmon begin to brown.

Nutrition Info: Calories: 89, Sodium: 133 mg, Dietary Fiber: 2.0 g, Total Fat: 1.1 g, Total Carbs: 16.5 g, Protein: 3.8 g.

107.Herb-roasted Turkey Breast

Servings: 8
Cooking Time: 60 Minutes
Ingredients:
- 3 lb turkey breast
- Rub Ingredients:
- 2 tbsp olive oil
- 2 tbsp lemon juice
- 1 tbsp minced Garlic
- 2 tsp ground mustard
- 2 tsp kosher salt
- 1 tsp pepper
- 1 tsp dried rosemary
- 1 tsp dried thyme
- 1 tsp ground sage

Directions:
1. Take a small bowl and thoroughly combine the Rub Ingredients: in it. Rub this on the outside of the turkey breast and under any loose skin.
2. Place the coated turkey breast keeping skin side up on a cooking tray.
3. Place the drip pan at the bottom of the cooking chamber of the Instant Pot Duo Crisp Air Fryer. Select Air Fry option, post this, adjust the temperature to 360°F and the time to one hour, then touch start.
4. When preheated, add the food to the cooking tray in the lowest position. Close the lid for cooking.
5. When the Air Fry program is complete, check to make sure that the thickest portion of the meat reads at least 160°F, remove the turkey and let it rest for 10 minutes before slicing and serving.

Nutrition Info: Calories 214, Total Fat 10g, Total Carbs 2g, Protein 29g

108.Parmesan Chicken Meatballs

Servings: 4
Cooking Time: 12 Minutes
Ingredients:
- 1-lb. ground chicken
- 1 large egg, beaten
- ½ cup Parmesan cheese, grated
- ½ cup pork rinds, ground
- 1 teaspoon garlic powder
- 1 teaspoon paprika
- 1 teaspoon kosher salt
- ½ teaspoon pepper
- Crust:
- ½ cup pork rinds, ground

Directions:
1. Toss all the meatball Ingredients: in a bowl and mix well.
2. Make small meatballs out this mixture and roll them in the pork rinds.
3. Place the coated meatballs in the air fryer basket.
4. Press "Power Button" of Air Fry Oven and turn the dial to select the "Bake" mode.
5. Press the Time button and again turn the dial to set the cooking time to 12 minutes.
6. Now push the Temp button and rotate the dial to set the temperature at 400 degrees F.
7. Once preheated, place the air fryer basket inside and close its lid.
8. Serve warm.

Nutrition Info: Calories 529 Total Fat 17 g Saturated Fat 3 g Cholesterol 65 mg Sodium 391 mg Total Carbs 55 g Fiber 6 g Sugar 8 g Protein 41g

109.Tomato Frittata

Servings: 2
Cooking Time: 30 Minutes
Ingredients:
- 4 eggs
- ¼ cup onion, chopped
- ½ cup tomatoes, chopped
- ½ cup milk
- 1 cup Gouda cheese, shredded
- Salt, as required

Directions:
1. In a small baking pan, add all the ingredients and mix well.
2. Press "Power Button" of Air Fry Oven and turn the dial to select the "Air Fry" mode.
3. Press the Time button and again turn the dial to set the cooking time to 30 minutes.
4. Now push the Temp button and rotate the dial to set the temperature at 340 degrees F.
5. Press "Start/Pause" button to start.
6. When the unit beeps to show that it is preheated, open the lid.
7. Arrange the baking pan over the "Wire Rack" and insert in the oven.
8. Cut into 2 wedges and serve.

Nutrition Info: Calories: 247 Cal Total Fat: 16.1 g Saturated Fat: 7.5 g Cholesterol: 332 mg Sodium: 417 mg Total Carbs: 7.30 g Fiber: 0.9 g Sugar: 5.2 g Protein: 18.6 g

110.Fried Chicken Tacos

Servings: 4
Cooking Time: 10 Minutes
Ingredients:
- Chicken
- 1 lb. chicken tenders or breast chopped into 2-inch pieces
- 1 tsp garlic powder
- ½ tsp onion powder
- 1 large egg
- 1 ½ tsp salt
- 1 tsp paprika
- 3 Tbsp buttermilk
- ¾ cup All-purpose flour
- 3 Tbsp corn starch
- ½ tsp black pepper
- ½ tsp cayenne pepper
- oil for spraying
- Coleslaw
- ¼ tsp red pepper flakes
- 2 cups coleslaw mix
- 1 Tbsp brown sugar
- ½ tsp salt
- 2 Tbsp apple cider vinegar
- 1 Tbsp water
- Spicy Mayo
- ½ tsp salt
- ¼ cup mayonnaise
- 1 tsp garlic powder
- 2 Tbsp hot sauce
- 1 Tbsp buttermilk
- Tortilla wrappers

Directions:
1. Take a large bowl and mix together coleslaw mix, water, brown sugar, salt, apple cider vinegar, and red pepper flakes. Set aside.
2. Take another small bowl and combine mayonnaise, hot sauce, buttermilk, garlic powder, and salt. Set this mixture aside.
3. Select the Instant Pot Duo Crisp Air Fryer option, adjust the temperature to 360°F and push start. Preheating will start.
4. Create a clear station by placing two large flat pans side by side. Whisk together egg and buttermilk with salt and pepper in one of them. In the second, whisk flour, corn starch, black pepper, garlic powder, onion powder, salt, paprika, and cayenne pepper.
5. Cut the chicken tenders into 1-inch pieces. Season all pieces with a little salt and pepper.
6. Once the Instant Pot Duo Crisp Air Fryer is preheated, remove the tray and lightly spray it with oil. Coat your chicken with egg mixture while shaking off any excess egg, followed by the flour mixture, and place it on the tray and tray in the basket, making sure your chicken pieces don't overlap.
7. Close the Air Fryer lid, and cook on 360°F for 10 minutes
8. while flipping and spraying halfway through cooking.
9. Once the chicken is done, remove and place chicken into warmed tortilla shells. Top with coleslaw and spicy mayonnaise.

Nutrition Info: Calories 375, Total Fat 15g, Total Carbs 31g, Protein 29g

111.Squash And Zucchini Mini Pizza

Servings: 4
Cooking Time: 15 Minutes
Ingredients:
- 1 pizza crust
- 1/2 cup parmesan cheese
- 4 tablespoons oregano
- 1 zucchini
- 1 yellow summer squash
- Olive oil
- Salt and pepper

Directions:
1. Start by preheating toaster oven to 350°F.

2. If you are using homemade crust, roll out 8 mini portions; if crust is store-bought, use a cookie cutter to cut out the portions.
3. Sprinkle parmesan and oregano equally on each piece. Layer the zucchini and squash in a circle – one on top of the other – around the entire circle.
4. Brush with olive oil and sprinkle salt and pepper to taste.
5. Bake for 15 minutes and serve.
Nutrition Info: Calories: 151, Sodium: 327 mg, Dietary Fiber: 3.1 g, Total Fat: 8.6 g, Total Carbs: 10.3 g, Protein: 11.4 g.

112. Roasted Grape And Goat Cheese Crostinis

Servings: 10
Cooking Time: 5 Minutes
Ingredients:
- 1 pound seedless red grapes
- 1 teaspoon chopped rosemary
- 4 tablespoons olive oil
- 1 rustic French baguette
- 1 cup sliced shallots
- 2 tablespoons unsalted butter
- 8 ounces goat cheese
- 1 tablespoon honey

Directions:
1. Start by preheating toaster oven to 400°F.
2. Toss grapes, rosemary, and 1 tablespoon of olive oil in a large bowl.
3. Transfer to a roasting pan and roast for 20 minutes.
4. Remove the pan from the oven and set aside to cool.
5. Slice the baguette into 1/2-inch-thick pieces.
6. Brush each slice with olive oil and place on baking sheet.
7. Bake for 8 minutes, then remove from oven and set aside.
8. In a medium skillet add butter and one tablespoon of olive oil.
9. Add shallots and sauté for about 10 minutes.
10. Mix goat cheese and honey in a medium bowl, then add contents of shallot pan and mix thoroughly.
11. Spread shallot mixture onto baguette, top with grapes, and serve.
Nutrition Info: Calories: 238, Sodium: 139 mg, Dietary Fiber: 0.6 g, Total Fat: 16.3 g, Total Carbs: 16.4 g, Protein: 8.4 g.

113. Balsamic Roasted Chicken

Servings: 4

Cooking Time: 1 Hour
Ingredients:
- 1/2 cup balsamic vinegar
- 1/4 cup Dijon mustard
- 1/3 cup olive oil
- Juice and zest from 1 lemon
- 3 minced garlic cloves
- 1 teaspoon salt
- 1 teaspoon pepper
- 4 bone-in, skin-on chicken thighs
- 4 bone-in, skin-on chicken drumsticks
- 1 tablespoon chopped parsley

Directions:
1. Mix vinegar, lemon juice, mustard, olive oil, garlic, salt, and pepper in a bowl, then pour into a sauce pan.
2. Roll chicken pieces in the pan, then cover and marinate for at least 2 hours, but up to 24 hours.
3. Preheat the toaster oven to 400°F and place the chicken on a fresh baking sheet, reserving the marinade for later.
4. Roast the chicken for 50 minutes.
5. Remove the chicken and cover it with foil to keep it warm. Place the marinade in the toaster oven for about 5 minutes until it simmers down and begins to thicken.
6. Pour marinade over chicken and sprinkle with parsley and lemon zest.
Nutrition Info: Calories: 1537, Sodium: 1383 mg, Dietary Fiber: 0.8 g, Total Fat: 70.5 g, Total Carbs: 2.4 g, Protein: 210.4 g.

114. Buttery Artichokes

Servings: 4
Cooking Time: 20 Minutes
Ingredients:
- 4 artichokes, trimmed and halved
- 3 garlic cloves, minced
- 1 tablespoon olive oil
- Salt and black pepper to the taste
- 4 tablespoons butter, melted
- ¼ teaspoon cumin, ground
- 1 tablespoon lemon zest, grated

Directions:
1. In a bowl, combine the artichokes with the oil, garlic and the other Ingredients:, toss well and transfer them to the air fryer's basket.
2. Cook for 20 minutes at 370 degrees F, divide between plates and serve as a side dish.
Nutrition Info: Calories 214, fat 5, fiber 8, carbs 12, protein 5

DINNER RECIPES

115. Kale And Brussels Sprouts

Servings: 8
Cooking Time: 7 Minutes
Ingredients:
- 1 lb. Brussels sprouts, trimmed
- 3 oz. mozzarella, shredded
- 2 cups kale, torn
- 1 tbsp. olive oil
- Salt and black pepper to taste.

Directions:
1. In a pan that fits the air fryer, combine all the Ingredients: except the mozzarella and toss.
2. Put the pan in the air fryer and cook at 380°F for 15 minutes
3. Divide between plates, sprinkle the cheese on top and serve.

Nutrition Info: Calories: 170; Fat: 5g; Fiber: 3g; Carbs: 4g; Protein: 7g

116. Salmon Steak Grilled With Cilantro Garlic Sauce

Servings: 2
Cooking Time: 15 Minutes
Ingredients:
- 2 salmon steaks
- Salt and pepper to taste
- 2 tablespoons vegetable oil
- 2 cloves of garlic, minced
- 1 cup cilantro leaves
- ½ cup Greek yogurt
- 1 teaspoon honey

Directions:
1. Place the instant pot air fryer lid on and preheat the instant pot at 390 degrees F.
2. Place the grill pan accessory in the instant pot.
3. Season the salmon steaks with salt and pepper. Brush with oil.
4. Place on the grill pan, close the air fryer lid and grill for 15 minutes and make sure to flip halfway through the cooking time.
5. In a food processor, mix the garlic, cilantro leaves, yogurt, and honey. Season with salt and pepper to taste. Pulse until smooth.
6. Serve the salmon steaks with the cilantro sauce.

Nutrition Info: Calories: 485; Carbs: 6.3g; Protein: 47.6g; Fat: 29.9g

117. Beef, Mushrooms And Noodles Dish

Servings: 5
Cooking Time: 35 Minutes
Ingredients:

- 1½ pounds beef steak
- 1 package egg noodles, cooked
- 1 ounce dry onion soup mix
- 1 can (15 oz cream mushroom soup
- 2 cups mushrooms, sliced
- 1 whole onion, chopped
- ½ cup beef broth
- 3 garlic cloves, minced?

Directions:
1. Preheat your Air Fryer to 360 F. Drizzle onion soup mix all over the meat. In a mixing bowl, mix the sauce, garlic cloves, beef broth, chopped onion, sliced mushrooms and mushroom soup. Top the meat with the prepared sauce mixture. Place the prepared meat in the air fryer's cooking basket and cook for 25 minutes. Serve with cooked egg noodles.

Nutrition Info: 346 Calories; 11g Fat; 4g Carbs; 32g Protein; 1g Sugars; 1g Fiber

118. Green Beans And Lime Sauce

Servings: 4
Cooking Time: 20 Minutes
Ingredients:
- 1 lb. green beans, trimmed
- 2 tbsp. ghee; melted
- 1 tbsp. lime juice
- 1 tsp. chili powder
- A pinch of salt and black pepper

Directions:
1. Take a bowl and mix the ghee with the rest of the ingredients except the green beans and whisk really well.
2. Mix the green beans with the lime sauce, toss
3. Put them in your air fryer's basket and cook at 400°F for 8 minutes. Serve right away.

Nutrition Info: Calories: 151; Fat: 4g; Fiber: 2g; Carbs: 4g; Protein: 6g

119. Lamb Skewers

Servings: 4
Cooking Time: 20 Minutes
Ingredients:
- 2 lb. lamb meat; cubed
- 2 red bell peppers; cut into medium pieces
- ¼ cup olive oil
- 2 tbsp. lemon juice
- 1 tbsp. oregano; dried
- 1 tbsp. red vinegar
- 1 tbsp. garlic; minced
- ½ tsp. rosemary; dried
- A pinch of salt and black pepper

Directions:

1. Take a bowl and mix all the ingredients and toss them well.
2. Thread the lamb and bell peppers on skewers, place them in your air fryer's basket and cook at 380°F for 10 minutes on each side. Divide between plates and serve with a side salad
Nutrition Info: Calories: 274; Fat: 12g; Fiber: 3g; Carbs: 6g; Protein: 16g

120. Tasty Grilled Red Mullet

Servings: 8
Cooking Time: 15 Minutes
Ingredients:
- 8 whole red mullets, gutted and scales removed
- Salt and pepper to taste
- Juice from 1 lemon
- 1 tablespoon olive oil

Directions:
1. Place the instant pot air fryer lid on and preheat the instant pot at 390 degrees F.
2. Place the grill pan accessory in the instant pot.
3. Season the red mullet with salt, pepper, and lemon juice.
4. Place red mullets on the grill pan and brush with olive oil.
5. Close the air fryer lid and grill for 15 minutes.
Nutrition Info: Calories: 152; Carbs: 0.9g; Protein: 23.1g; Fat: 6.2g

121. Green Beans And Mushroom Casserole

Servings: 6
Cooking Time: 12 Minutes
Ingredients:
- 24 ounces fresh green beans, trimmed
- 2 cups fresh button mushrooms, sliced
- 1/3 cup French fried onions
- 3 tablespoons olive oil
- 2 tablespoons fresh lemon juice
- 1 teaspoon ground sage
- 1 teaspoon garlic powder
- 1 teaspoon onion powder
- Salt and black pepper, to taste

Directions:
1. Preheat the Air fryer to 400F and grease an Air fryer basket.
2. Mix the green beans, mushrooms, oil, lemon juice, sage, and spices in a bowl and toss to coat well.
3. Arrange the green beans mixture into the Air fryer basket and cook for about 12 minutes.
4. Dish out in a serving dish and top with fried onions to serve.

Nutrition Info: Calories: 65, Fat: 1.6g, Carbohydrates: 11g, Sugar: 2.4g, Protein: 3g, Sodium: 52mg

122. Coconut Crusted Shrimp

Servings: 3
Cooking Time: 40 Minutes
Ingredients:
- 8 ounces coconut milk
- ½ cup sweetened coconut, shredded
- ½ cup panko breadcrumbs
- 1 pound large shrimp, peeled and deveined
- Salt and black pepper, to taste

Directions:
1. Preheat the Air fryer to 350-degree F and grease an Air fryer basket.
2. Place the coconut milk in a shallow bowl.
3. Mix coconut, breadcrumbs, salt, and black pepper in another bowl.
4. Dip each shrimp into coconut milk and finally, dredge in the coconut mixture.
5. Arrange half of the shrimps into the Air fryer basket and cook for about 20 minutes.
6. Dish out the shrimps onto serving plates and repeat with the remaining mixture to serve.
Nutrition Info: Calories: 408, Fats: 23.7g, Carbohydrates: 11.7g, Sugar: 3.4g, Proteins: 31g, Sodium: 253mg

123. Cheesy Shrimp

Servings: 4
Cooking Time: 20 Minutes
Ingredients:
- 2/3 cup Parmesan cheese, grated
- 2 pounds shrimp, peeled and deveined
- 4 garlic cloves, minced
- 2 tablespoons olive oil
- 1 teaspoon dried basil
- ½ teaspoon dried oregano
- 1 teaspoon onion powder
- ½ teaspoon red pepper flakes, crushed
- Ground black pepper, as required
- 2 tablespoons fresh lemon juice

Directions:
1. Preheat the Air fryer to 350 degree F and grease an Air fryer basket.
2. Mix Parmesan cheese, garlic, olive oil, herbs, and spices in a large bowl.
3. Arrange half of the shrimp into the Air fryer basket in a single layer and cook for about 10 minutes.
4. Dish out the shrimps onto serving plates and drizzle with lemon juice to serve hot.

Nutrition Info: Calories: 386, Fat: 14.2g, Carbohydrates: 5.3g, Sugar: 0.4g, Protein: 57.3g, Sodium: 670mg

124.Fish Cakes With Horseradish Sauce

Servings: 4
Cooking Time: 20 Minutes
Ingredients:
- Halibut Cakes:
- 1 pound halibut
- 2 tablespoons olive oil
- 1/2 teaspoon cayenne pepper
- 1/4 teaspoon black pepper
- Salt, to taste
- 2 tablespoons cilantro, chopped
- 1 shallot, chopped
- 2 garlic cloves, minced
- 1 cup Romano cheese, grated
- 1 egg, whisked
- 1 tablespoon Worcestershire sauce
- Mayo Sauce:
- 1 teaspoon horseradish, grated
- 1/2 cup mayonnaise

Directions:
1. Start by preheating your Air Fryer to 380 degrees F. Spritz the Air Fryer basket with cooking oil.
2. Mix all ingredients for the halibut cakes in a bowl; knead with your hands until everything is well incorporated.
3. Shape the mixture into equally sized patties. Transfer your patties to the Air Fryer basket. Cook the fish patties for 10 minutes, turning them over halfway through.
4. Mix the horseradish and mayonnaise. Serve the halibut cakes with the horseradish mayo.

Nutrition Info: 532 Calories; 32g Fat; 3g Carbs; 28g Protein; 3g Sugars; 6g Fiber

125.Healthy Mama Meatloaf

Servings: 8
Cooking Time: 40 Minutes
Ingredients:
- 1 tablespoon olive oil
- 1 green bell pepper, diced
- 1/2 cup diced sweet onion
- 1/2 teaspoon minced garlic
- 1-lb. ground beef
- 1 cup whole wheat bread crumbs
- 2 large eggs
- 3/4 cup shredded carrot
- 3/4 cup shredded zucchini
- salt and ground black pepper to taste

- 1/4 cup ketchup, or to taste

Directions:
1. Thoroughly mix ground beef with egg, onion, garlic, crumbs, and all the ingredients in a bowl.
2. Grease a meatloaf pan with oil or butter and spread the minced beef in the pan.
3. Press "Power Button" of Air Fry Oven and turn the dial to select the "Bake" mode.
4. Press the Time button and again turn the dial to set the cooking time to 40 minutes.
5. Now push the Temp button and rotate the dial to set the temperature at 375 degrees F.
6. Once preheated, place the beef baking pan in the oven and close its lid.
7. Slice and serve.

Nutrition Info: Calories: 322 Cal Total Fat: 11.8 g Saturated Fat: 2.2 g Cholesterol: 56 mg Sodium: 321 mg Total Carbs: 14.6 g Fiber: 4.4 g Sugar: 8 g Protein: 17.3 g

126.Air Fryer Buffalo Mushroom Poppers

Servings: 8
Cooking Time: 50 Minutes
Ingredients:
- 1 pound fresh whole button mushrooms
- 1/2 teaspoon kosher salt
- 3 tablespoons 1/3-less-fat cream cheese,
- 1/4 cup all-purpose flour
- Softened 1 jalapeño chile, seeded and minced
- Cooking spray
- 1/4 teaspoon black pepper
- 1 cup panko breadcrumbs
- 2 large eggs, lightly beaten
- 1/4 cup buffalo-style hot sauce
- 2 tablespoons chopped fresh chives
- 1/2 cup low-fat buttermilk
- 1/2 cup plain fat-free yogurt
- 2 ounces blue cheese, crumbled (about 1/2 cup)
- 3 tablespoons apple cider vinegar

Directions:
1. Remove stems from mushroom caps, chop stems and set caps aside. Stir together chopped mushroom stems, cream cheese, jalapeño, salt, and pepper. Stuff about 1 teaspoon of the mixture into each mushroom cap, rounding the filling to form a smooth ball.
2. Place panko in a bowl, place flour in a second bowl, and eggs in a third Coat mushrooms in flour, dip in egg mixture, and dredge in panko, pressing to adhere. Spray mushrooms well with cooking spray.
3. Place half of the mushrooms in air fryer basket, and cook for 20 minutes at 350°F. Transfer cooked mushrooms to a large bowl. Drizzle buffalo sauce over mushrooms; toss to coat then sprinkle with chives.

4. Stir buttermilk, yogurt, blue cheese, and cider vinegar in a small bowl. Serve mushroom poppers with blue cheese sauce.
Nutrition Info: Calories 133 Fat 4g Saturated fat 2g Unsaturated fat 2g Protein 7g Carbohydrate 16g Fiber 1g Sugars 3g Sodium 485mg Calcium 10% DV Potassium 7% DV

127.Miso-glazed Salmon

Servings: 4
Cooking Time: 5 Minutes
Ingredients:
- 1/4 cup red or white miso
- 1/3 cup sake
- 1 tablespoon soy sauce
- 2 tablespoons vegetable oil
- 1/4 cup sugar
- 4 skinless salmon filets

Directions:
1. In a shallow bowl, mix together the miso, sake, oil, soy sauce, and sugar.
2. Toss the salmon in the mixture until thoroughly coated on all sides.
3. Preheat your toaster oven to "high" on broil mode.
4. Place salmon in a broiling pan and broil until the top is well charred—about 5 minutes.
Nutrition Info: Calories: 401, Sodium: 315 mg, Dietary Fiber: 0 g, Total Fat: 19.2 g, Total Carbs: 14.1 g, Protein: 39.2 g.

128.Turkey Wontons With Garlic-parmesan Sauce

Servings: 8
Cooking Time: 20 Minutes
Ingredients:
- 8 ounces cooked turkey breasts, shredded 16 wonton wrappers
- 1½ tablespoons margarine, melted
- 1/3 cup cream cheese, room temperature 8 ounces Asiago cheese, shredded
- 3 tablespoons Parmesan cheese, grated
- 1 tsp. garlic powder
- Fine sea salt and freshly ground black pepper, to taste

Directions:
1. In a small-sized bowl, mix the margarine, Parmesan, garlic powder, salt, and black pepper; give it a good stir.
2. Lightly grease a mini muffin pan; lay 1 wonton wrapper in each mini muffin cup. Fill each cup with the cream cheese and turkey mixture.

3. Air-fry for 8 minutes at 335 °F. Immediately top with Asiago cheese and serve warm.
Nutrition Info: 362 Calories; 13.5g Fat; 40.4g Carbs; 18.5g Protein; 1.2g Sugars

129.Artichoke Spinach Casserole

Servings: 4
Cooking Time: 20 Minutes
Ingredients:
- ⅓cup full-fat mayonnaise
- oz. full-fat cream cheese; softened.
- ¼ cup diced yellow onion
- ⅓cup full-fat sour cream.
- ¼ cup chopped pickled jalapeños.
- 2 cups fresh spinach; chopped
- 2 cups cauliflower florets; chopped
- 1 cup artichoke hearts; chopped
- 1 tbsp. salted butter; melted.

Directions:
1. Take a large bowl, mix butter, onion, cream cheese, mayonnaise and sour cream. Fold in jalapeños, spinach, cauliflower and artichokes.
2. Pour the mixture into a 4-cup round baking dish. Cover with foil and place into the air fryer basket
3. Adjust the temperature to 370 Degrees F and set the timer for 15 minutes. In the last 2 minutes of cooking, remove the foil to brown the top. Serve warm.
Nutrition Info: Calories: 423; Protein: 7g; Fiber: 3g; Fat: 33g; Carbs: 11g

130.Roasted Garlic Zucchini Rolls

Servings: 4
Cooking Time: 20 Minutes
Ingredients:
- 2 medium zucchinis
- ½ cup full-fat ricotta cheese
- ¼ white onion; peeled. And diced
- 2 cups spinach; chopped
- ¼ cup heavy cream
- ½ cup sliced baby portobello mushrooms
- ¾ cup shredded mozzarella cheese, divided.
- 2 tbsp. unsalted butter.
- 2 tbsp. vegetable broth.
- ½ tsp. finely minced roasted garlic
- ¼ tsp. dried oregano.
- ⅛ tsp. xanthan gum
- ¼ tsp. salt
- ½ tsp. garlic powder.

Directions:
1. Using a mandoline or sharp knife, slice zucchini into long strips lengthwise. Place strips between paper towels to absorb moisture. Set aside

2. In a medium saucepan over medium heat, melt butter. Add onion and sauté until fragrant. Add garlic and sauté 30 seconds.
3. Pour in heavy cream, broth and xanthan gum. Turn off heat and whisk mixture until it begins to thicken, about 3 minutes.
4. Take a medium bowl, add ricotta, salt, garlic powder and oregano and mix well. Fold in spinach, mushrooms and ½ cup mozzarella.
5. Pour half of the sauce into a 6-inch round baking pan. To assemble the rolls, place two strips of zucchini on a work surface. Spoon 2 tbsp. of ricotta mixture onto the slices and roll up. Place seam side down on top of sauce. Repeat with remaining ingredients
6. Pour remaining sauce over the rolls and sprinkle with remaining mozzarella. Cover with foil and place into the air fryer basket. Adjust the temperature to 350 Degrees F and set the timer for 20 minutes. In the last 5 minutes, remove the foil to brown the cheese. Serve immediately.
Nutrition Info: Calories: 245; Protein: 15g; Fiber: 8g; Fat: 19g; Carbs: 1g

131.Red Wine Infused Mushrooms

Servings: 6
Cooking Time: 30 Minutes
Ingredients:
- 1 tablespoon butter
- 2 pounds fresh mushrooms, quartered
- 2 teaspoons Herbs de Provence
- ½ teaspoon garlic powder
- 2 tablespoons red wine

Directions:
1. Preheat the Air fryer to 325F and grease an Air fryer pan.
2. Mix the butter, Herbs de Provence, and garlic powder in the Air fryer pan and toss to coat well.
3. Cook for about 2 minutes and stir in the mushrooms and red wine.
4. Cook for about 28 minutes and dish out in a platter to serve hot.
Nutrition Info: Calories: 54, Fat: 2.4g, Carbohydrates: 5.3g, Sugar: 2.7g, Protein: 4.8g, Sodium: 23mg

132.Corned Beef With Carrots

Servings: 3
Cooking Time: 35 Minutes
Ingredients:
- 1 tbsp beef spice
- 1 whole onion, chopped
- 4 carrots, chopped
- 12 oz bottle beer

- 1½ cups chicken broth
- 4 pounds corned beef

Directions:
1. Preheat your air fryer to 380 f. Cover beef with beer and set aside for 20 minutes. Place carrots, onion and beef in a pot and heat over high heat. Add in broth and bring to a boil. Drain boiled meat and veggies; set aside.
2. Top with beef spice. Place the meat and veggies in your air fryer's cooking basket and cook for 30 minutes.
Nutrition Info: Calories: 464 Cal Total Fat: 17 g Saturated Fat: 6.8 g Cholesterol: 91.7 mg Sodium: 1904.2 mg Total Carbs: 48.9 g Fiber: 7.2 g Sugar: 5.8 g Protein: 30.6 g

133.Asparagus Frittata

Servings: 4
Cooking Time: 10 Minutes
Ingredients:
- 6 eggs
- 3 mushrooms, sliced
- 10 asparagus, chopped 1/4 cup half and half
- 2 tsp butter, melted
- 1 cup mozzarella cheese, shredded 1 tsp pepper
- 1 tsp salt

Directions:
1. Toss mushrooms and asparagus with melted butter and add into the air fryer basket.
2. Cook mushrooms and asparagus at 350 F for 5 minutes. Shake basket twice.
3. Meanwhile, in a bowl, whisk together eggs, half and half, pepper, and salt.
4. Transfer cook mushrooms and asparagus into the air fryer baking dish.
5. Pour egg mixture over mushrooms and asparagus.
6. Place dish in the air fryer and cook at 350 F for 5 minutes or until eggs are set.
7. Slice and serve.
Nutrition Info: Calories 211 Fat 13 g Carbohydrates 4 g Sugar 1 g Protein 16 g Cholesterol 272 mg

134.Cheese Zucchini Boats

Servings: 2
Cooking Time: 20 Minutes
Ingredients:
- 2 medium zucchinis
- ¼ cup full-fat ricotta cheese
- ¼ cup shredded mozzarella cheese
- ¼ cup low-carb, no-sugar-added pasta sauce.
- 2 tbsp. grated vegetarian Parmesan cheese
- 1 tbsp. avocado oil

- ¼ tsp. garlic powder.
- ½ tsp. dried parsley.
- ¼ tsp. dried oregano.

Directions:
1. Cut off 1-inch from the top and bottom of each zucchini.
2. Slice zucchini in half lengthwise and use a spoon to scoop out a bit of the inside, making room for filling. Brush with oil and spoon 2 tbsp. pasta sauce into each shell
3. Take a medium bowl, mix ricotta, mozzarella, oregano, garlic powder and parsley
4. Spoon the mixture into each zucchini shell. Place stuffed zucchini shells into the air fryer basket.
5. Adjust the temperature to 350 Degrees F and set the timer for 20 minutes
6. To remove from the fryer basket, use tongs or a spatula and carefully lift out. Top with Parmesan. Serve immediately.

Nutrition Info: Calories: 215; Protein: 15g; Fiber: 7g; Fat: 19g; Carbs: 3g

135.Zucchini Muffins

Servings: 8
Cooking Time: 20 Minutes
Ingredients:
- 6 eggs
- 4 drops stevia 1/4 cup Swerve
- 1/3 cup coconut oil, melted 1 cup zucchini, grated
- 3/4 cup coconut flour 1/4 tsp ground nutmeg 1 tsp ground cinnamon 1/2 tsp baking soda

Directions:
1. Preheat the air fryer to 325 F.
2. Add all ingredients except zucchini in a bowl and mix well.
3. Add zucchini and stir well.
4. Pour batter into the silicone muffin molds and place into the air fryer basket.
5. Cook muffins for 20 minutes.
6. Serve and enjoy.

Nutrition Info: Calories 136 Fat 12 g Carbohydrates 1 g Sugar 0.6 g Protein 4 g Cholesterol 123 mg

136.Shrimp Casserole Louisiana Style

Servings: 2
Cooking Time: 35 Minutes
Ingredients:
- 3/4 cup uncooked instant rice
- 3/4 cup water
- 1/2 pound small shrimp, peeled and deveined
- 1 tablespoon butter
- 1/2 (4 ounces) can sliced mushrooms, drained

- 1/2 (8 ounces) container sour cream
- 1/3 cup shredded Cheddar cheese

Directions:
1. Place the instant pot air fryer lid on, lightly grease baking pan of the instant pot with cooking spray. Add rice, water, mushrooms, and butter. Cover with foil and place the baking pan in the instant pot.
2. Close the air fryer lid and cook at 360F for 20 minutes.
3. Open foil cover, stir in shrimps, return foil and let it rest for 5 minutes.
4. Remove foil completely and stir in sour cream. Mix well and evenly spread rice. Top with cheese.
5. Cook for 7 minutes at 390F until tops are lightly browned.
6. Serve and enjoy.

Nutrition Info: Calories: 569; Carbs: 38.5g; Protein: 31.8g; Fat: 31.9g

137.Air Fryer Veggie Quesdillas

Servings: 4
Cooking Time: 40 Minutes
Ingredients:
- 4 sprouted whole-grain flour tortillas (6-in.)
- 1 cup sliced red bell pepper
- 4 ounces reduced-fat Cheddar cheese, shredded
- 1 cup sliced zucchini
- 1 cup canned black beans, drained and rinsed (no salt)
- Cooking spray
- 2 ounces plain 2% reduced-fat Greek yogurt
- 1 teaspoon lime zest
- 1 Tbsp. fresh juice (from 1 lime)
- ¼ tsp. ground cumin
- 2 tablespoons chopped fresh cilantro
- 1/2 cup drained refrigerated pico de gallo

Directions:
1. Place tortillas on work surface, sprinkle 2 tablespoons shredded cheese over half of each tortilla and top with cheese on each tortilla with 1/4 cup each red pepper slices, zucchini slices, and black beans. Sprinkle evenly with remaining 1/2 cup cheese.
2. Fold tortillas over to form half-moon shaped quesadillas, lightly coat with cooking spray, and secure with toothpicks.
3. Lightly spray air fryer basket with cooking spray. Place 2 quesadillas in the basket, and cook at 400°F for 10 minutes until tortillas are golden brown and slightly crispy, cheese is melted, and vegetables are slightly softened. Turn quesadillas over halfway through cooking.
4. Repeat with remaining quesadillas.
5. Meanwhile, stir yogurt, lime juice, lime zest and cumin in a small bowl.

6. Cut each quesadilla into wedges and sprinkle with cilantro.
7. Serve with 1 tablespoon cumin cream and 2 tablespoons pico de gallo each.
Nutrition Info: Calories 291 Fat 8g Saturated fat 4g Unsaturated fat 3g Protein 17g Carbohydrate 36g Fiber 8g Sugars 3g Sodium 518mg Calcium 30% DV Potassium 6% DV

138.Grilled Tasty Scallops

Servings: 2
Cooking Time: 10 Minutes
Ingredients:
- 1 pound sea scallops, cleaned and patted dry
- Salt and pepper to taste
- 3 dried chilies
- 2 tablespoon dried thyme
- 1 tablespoon dried oregano
- 1 tablespoon ground coriander
- 1 tablespoon ground fennel
- 2 teaspoons chipotle pepper

Directions:
1. Place the instant pot air fryer lid on and preheat the instant pot at 390 degrees F.
2. Place the grill pan accessory in the instant pot.
3. Mix all ingredients in a bowl.
4. Dump the scallops on the grill pan, close the air fryer lid and cook for 10 minutes.
Nutrition Info: Calories:291 ; Carbs: 20.7g; Protein: 48.6g; Fat: 2.5g

139.Beef Roast

Servings: 4
Ingredients:
- 2 lbs. beef roast
- 1 tbsp. smoked paprika
- 3 tbsp. garlic; minced
- 3 tbsp. olive oil
- Salt and black pepper to taste

Directions:
1. In a bowl, combine all the ingredients and coat the roast well.
2. Place the roast in your air fryer and cook at 390°F for 55 minutes. Slice the roast, divide it between plates and serve with a side salad

140.Shrimp Kebabs

Servings: 2
Cooking Time: 10 Minutes
Ingredients:
- ¾ pound shrimp, peeled and deveined
- 1 tablespoon fresh cilantro, chopped

- Wooden skewers, presoaked
- 2 tablespoons fresh lemon juice
- 1 teaspoon garlic, minced
- ½ teaspoon paprika
- ½ teaspoon ground cumin
- Salt and ground black pepper, as required

Directions:
1. Preheat the Air fryer to 350 degree F and grease an Air fryer basket.
2. Mix lemon juice, garlic, and spices in a bowl.
3. Stir in the shrimp and mix to coat well.
4. Thread the shrimp onto presoaked wooden skewers and transfer to the Air fryer basket.
5. Cook for about 10 minutes, flipping once in between.
6. Dish out the mixture onto serving plates and serve garnished with fresh cilantro.
Nutrition Info: Calories: 212, Fat: 3.2g, Carbohydrates: 3.9g, Sugar: 0.4g, Protein: 39.1g, Sodium: 497mg

141.Baby Portabellas With Romano Cheese

Servings: 4
Cooking Time: 20 Minutes
Ingredients:
- 1 pound baby portabellas
- 1/2 cup almond meal
- 2 eggs
- 2 tablespoons milk
- 1 cup Romano cheese, grated
- Sea salt and ground black pepper
- 1/2 teaspoon shallot powder
- 1 teaspoon garlic powder
- 1/2 teaspoon cumin powder
- 1/2 teaspoon cayenne pepper

Directions:
1. Pat the mushrooms dry with a paper towel.
2. To begin, set up your breading station. Place the almond meal in a shallow dish. In a separate dish, whisk the eggs with milk.
3. Finally, place grated Romano cheese and seasonings in the third dish.
4. Start by dredging the baby portabellas in the almond meal mixture; then, dip them into the egg wash. Press the baby portabellas into Romano cheese, coating evenly.
5. Spritz the Air Fryer basket with cooking oil. Add the baby portabellas and cook at 400 degrees F for 6 minutes, flipping them halfway through the cooking time.
Nutrition Info: 230 Calories; 13g Fat; 2g Carbs; 11g Protein; 8g Sugars; 6g Fiber

142.Garlic Lamb Shank

Servings: 5
Cooking Time: 24 Minutes
Ingredients:
- 17 oz. lamb shanks
- 2 tablespoon garlic, peeled
- 1 teaspoon kosher salt
- 1 tablespoon dried parsley
- 4 oz chive stems, chopped
- ½ cup chicken stock
- 1 teaspoon butter
- 1 teaspoon dried rosemary
- 1 teaspoon nutmeg
- ½ teaspoon ground black pepper

Directions:
1. Chop the garlic roughly.
2. Make the cuts in the lamb shank and fill the cuts with the chopped garlic.
3. Then sprinkle the lamb shank with the kosher salt, dried parsley, dried rosemary, nutmeg, and ground black pepper.
4. Stir the spices on the lamb shank gently.
5. Then put the butter and chicken stock in the air fryer basket tray.
6. Preheat the air fryer to 380 F.
7. Put the chives in the air fryer basket tray.
8. Add the lamb shank and cook the meat for 24 minutes.
9. When the lamb shank is cooked – transfer it to the serving plate and sprinkle with the remaining liquid from the cooked meat.
10. Enjoy!

Nutrition Info: calories 205, fat 8.2, fiber 0.8, carbs 3.8, protein 27.2

143.Cheddar Pork Meatballs

Servings: 4 To 6
Cooking Time: 25 Minutes
Ingredients:
- 1 lb ground pork
- 1 large onion, chopped
- ½ tsp maple syrup
- 2 tsp mustard
- ½ cup chopped basil leaves
- Salt and black pepper to taste
- 2 tbsp. grated cheddar cheese

Directions:
1. In a mixing bowl, add the ground pork, onion, maple syrup, mustard, basil leaves, salt, pepper, and cheddar cheese; mix well. Use your hands to form bite-size balls. Place in the fryer basket and cook at 400 f for 10 minutes.
2. Slide out the fryer basket and shake it to toss the meatballs. Cook further for 5 minutes. Remove them

onto a wire rack and serve with zoodles and marinara sauce.

Nutrition Info: Calories: 300 Cal Total Fat: 24 g Saturated Fat: 9 g Cholesterol: 70 mg Sodium: 860 mg Total Carbs: 3 g Fiber: 0 g Sugar: 0 g Protein: 16 g

144.Fried Spicy Tofu

Servings: 4
Cooking Time: 20 Minutes
Ingredients:
- 16 ounces firm tofu, pressed and cubed
- 1 tablespoon vegan oyster sauce
- 1 tablespoon tamari sauce
- 1 teaspoon cider vinegar
- 1 teaspoon pure maple syrup
- 1 teaspoon sriracha
- 1/2 teaspoon shallot powder
- 1/2 teaspoon porcini powder
- 1 teaspoon garlic powder
- 1 tablespoon sesame oil
- 2 tablespoons golden flaxseed meal

Directions:
1. Toss the tofu with the oyster sauce, tamari sauce, vinegar,maple syrup, sriracha, shallot powder, porcini powder, garlic powder, and sesame oil. Let it marinate for 30 minutes.
2. Toss the marinated tofu with the flaxseed meal.
3. Cook at 360 degrees F for 10 minutes; turn them over and cook for 12 minutes more.

Nutrition Info: 173 Calories; 13g Fat; 5g Carbs; 12g Protein; 8g Sugars; 1g Fiber

145.Beef With Apples And Plums

Servings: 4
Cooking Time: 30 Minutes
Ingredients:
- 2pounds beef stew meat, cubed
- 1cup apples, cored and cubed
- 1cup plums, pitted and halved
- 2tablespoons butter, melted
- Salt and black pepper to the taste
- ½ cup red wine
- 1tablespoon chives, chopped

Directions:
1. In the air fryer's pan, mix the beef with the apples and the other ingredients, toss, put the pan in the machine and cook at 390 degrees F for 30 minutes.
2. Divide the mix between plates and serve right away.

Nutrition Info: Calories 290, Fat 12, Fiber 5, Carbs 19, Protein 28

146.Sautéed Green Beans

Servings: 2
Cooking Time: 10 Minutes
Ingredients:
- 8 ounces fresh green beans, trimmed and cut in half
- 1 teaspoon sesame oil
- 1 tablespoon soy sauce

Directions:
1. Preheat the Air fryer to 390F and grease an Air fryer basket.
2. Mix green beans, soy sauce, and sesame oil in a bowl and toss to coat well.
3. Arrange green beans into the Air fryer basket and cook for about 10 minutes, tossing once in between.
4. Dish out onto serving plates and serve hot.

Nutrition Info: Calories: 59, Fats: 2.4g, Carbohydrates: 59g, Sugar: 1.7g, Proteins: 2.6g, Sodium: 458mg

147.Stuffed Okra

Servings: 2
Cooking Time: 12 Minutes
Ingredients:
- 8 ounces large okra
- ¼ cup chickpea flour
- ¼ of onion, chopped
- 2 tablespoons coconut, grated freshly
- 1 teaspoon garam masala powder
- ½ teaspoon ground turmeric
- ½ teaspoon red chili powder
- ½ teaspoon ground cumin
- Salt, to taste

Directions:
1. Preheat the Air fryer to 390F and grease an Air fryer basket.
2. Mix the flour, onion, grated coconut, and spices in a bowl and toss to coat well.
3. Stuff the flour mixture into okra and arrange into the Air fryer basket.
4. Cook for about 12 minutes and dish out in a serving plate.

Nutrition Info: Calories: 166, Fat: 3.7g, Carbohydrates: 26.6g, Sugar: 5.3g, Protein: 7.6g, Sodium: 103mg

148.Air Fryer Roasted Broccoli

Servings: 4
Cooking Time: 10 Minutes
Ingredients:
- 1 tsp. herbes de provence seasoning (optional)
- 4 cups fresh broccoli
- 1 tablespoon olive oil
- Salt and pepper to taste

Directions:
1. Drizzle or spray broccoli with olive and sprinkle seasoning throughout
2. Spray air fryer basket with cooking oil, place broccoli and cook for 5-8 minutes on 360F
3. Open air fryer and examine broccoli after 5 minutes because different fryer brands cook at different rates.

Nutrition Info: Calories 61 Fat 4g protein 3g net carbs 4g

149.Tasty Sausage Bacon Rolls

Servings: 4
Cooking Time: 1 Hour 44 Minutes
Ingredients:
- Sausage:
- 8 bacon strips
- 8 pork sausages
- Relish:
- 8 large tomatoes
- 1 clove garlic, peeled
- 1 small onion, peeled
- 3 tbsp chopped parsley
- A pinch of salt
- A pinch of pepper
- 2 tbsp sugar
- 1 tsp smoked paprika
- 1 tbsp white wine vinegar

Directions:
1. Start with the relish; add the tomatoes, garlic, and onion in a food processor. Blitz them for 10 seconds until the mixture is pulpy. Pour the pulp into a saucepan, add the vinegar, salt, pepper, and place it over medium heat.
2. Bring to simmer for 10 minutes; add the paprika and sugar. Stir with a spoon and simmer for 10 minutes until pulpy and thick. Turn off the heat, transfer the relish to a bowl and chill it for an hour. In 30 minutes after putting the relish in the refrigerator, move on to the sausages. Wrap each sausage with a bacon strip neatly and stick in a bamboo skewer at the end of the sausage to secure the bacon ends.
3. Open the Air Fryer, place 3 to 4 wrapped sausages in the fryer basket and cook for 12 minutes at 350 F. Ensure that the bacon is golden and crispy before removing them. Repeat the cooking process for the remaining wrapped sausages. Remove the relish from the refrigerator. Serve the sausages and relish with turnip mash.

Nutrition Info: 346 Calories; 11g Fat; 4g Carbs; 32g Protein; 1g Sugars; 1g Fiber

150.Prawn Burgers

Servings: 2
Cooking Time: 6 Minutes
Ingredients:
- ½ cup prawns, peeled, deveined and finely chopped
- ½ cup breadcrumbs
- 2-3 tablespoons onion, finely chopped
- 3 cups fresh baby greens
- ½ teaspoon ginger, minced
- ½ teaspoon garlic, minced
- ½ teaspoon red chili powder
- ½ teaspoon ground cumin
- ¼ teaspoon ground turmeric
- Salt and ground black pepper, as required

Directions:
1. Preheat the Air fryer to 390 degree F and grease an Air fryer basket.
2. Mix the prawns, breadcrumbs, onion, ginger, garlic, and spices in a bowl.
3. Make small-sized patties from the mixture and transfer to the Air fryer basket.
4. Cook for about 6 minutes and dish out in a platter.
5. Serve immediately warm alongside the baby greens.

Nutrition Info: Calories: 240, Fat: 2.7g, Carbohydrates: 37.4g, Sugar: 4g, Protein: 18g, Sodium: 371mg

151.Cheddar & Dijon Tuna Melt

Servings: 1
Cooking Time: 7 Minutes
Ingredients:
- 1 (6-ounce) can tuna, drained and flaked
- 2 tablespoons mayonnaise
- 1 pinch salt
- 1 teaspoon balsamic vinegar
- 1 teaspoon Dijon mustard
- 2 slices whole wheat bread
- 2 teaspoons chopped dill pickle
- 1/4 cup shredded sharp cheddar cheese

Directions:
1. Start by preheating toaster oven to 375°F.
2. Put bread in toaster while it warms.
3. Mix together tuna, mayo, salt, vinegar, mustard, and pickle in a small bowl.
4. Remove bread from oven and put tuna mixture on one side and the cheese on the other.
5. Return to toaster oven and bake for 7 minutes.

6. Combine slices, then cut and serve.
Nutrition Info: Calories: 688, Sodium: 1024 mg, Dietary Fiber: 4.1 g, Total Fat: 35.0 g, Total Carbs: 31.0 g, Protein: 59.9 g.

152.Stuffed Potatoes

Servings: 4
Cooking Time: 31 Minutes
Ingredients:
- 4 potatoes, peeled
- 1 tablespoon butter
- ½ of brown onion, chopped
- 2 tablespoons chives, chopped
- ½ cup Parmesan cheese, grated
- 3 tablespoons canola oil

Directions:
1. Preheat the Air fryer to 390F and grease an Air fryer basket.
2. Coat the potatoes with canola oil and arrange into the Air fryer basket.
3. Cook for about 20 minutes and transfer into a platter.
4. Cut each potato in half and scoop out the flesh from each half.
5. Heat butter in a frying pan over medium heat and add onions.
6. Sauté for about 5 minutes and dish out in a bowl.
7. Mix the onions with the potato flesh, chives, and half of cheese.
8. Stir well and stuff the potato halves evenly with the onion potato mixture.
9. Top with the remaining cheese and arrange the potato halves into the Air fryer basket.
10. Cook for about 6 minutes and dish out to serve warm.

Nutrition Info: Calories: 328, Fat: 11.3g, Carbohydrates: 34.8g, Sugar: 3.1g, Protein: 5.8g, Sodium: 77mg

153.Pork Chops With Chicory Treviso

Servings: 2
Cooking Time: 0-15;
Ingredients:
- 4 pork chops
- 40g butter
- Flour to taste
- 1 chicory stalk
- Salt to taste

Directions:
1. Cut the chicory into small pieces. Place the butter and chicory in pieces on the basket of the air fryer previously preheated at 1800C and brown for 2 min.

2. Add the previously floured and salted pork slices (directly over the chicory), simmer for 6 minutes turning them over after 3 minutes.
3. Remove the slices and place them on a serving plate, covering them with the rest of the red chicory juice collected at the bottom of the basket.
Nutrition Info: Calories 504, Fat 33, Carbohydrates 0g, Sugars 0g, Protein 42g, Cholesterol 130mg

154.Crispy Scallops

Servings: 4
Cooking Time: 6 Minutes
Ingredients:
- 18 sea scallops, cleaned and patted very dry
- 1/8 cup all-purpose flour
- 1 tablespoon 2% milk
- ½ egg
- ¼ cup cornflakes, crushed
- ½ teaspoon paprika
- Salt and black pepper, as required

Directions:
1. Preheat the Air fryer to 400 degree F and grease an Air fryer basket.
2. Mix flour, paprika, salt, and black pepper in a bowl.
3. Whisk egg with milk in another bowl and place the cornflakes in a third bowl.
4. Coat each scallop with the flour mixture, dip into the egg mixture and finally, dredge in the cornflakes.
5. Arrange scallops in the Air fryer basket and cook for about 6 minutes.
6. Dish out the scallops in a platter and serve hot.
Nutrition Info: Calories: 150, Fat: 1.7g, Carbohydrates: 8g, Sugar: 0.4g, Protein: 24g, Sodium: 278mg

155.Sage Sausages Balls

Servings: 4
Cooking Time: 20 Minutes
Ingredients:
- 3 ½ oz sausages, sliced
- Salt and black pepper to taste
- 1 cup onion, chopped
- 3 tbsp breadcrumbs
- ½ tsp garlic puree
- 1 tsp sage

Directions:
1. Preheat your air fryer to 340 f. In a bowl, mix onions, sausage meat, sage, garlic puree, salt and pepper. Add breadcrumbs to a plate. Form balls using the mixture and roll them in breadcrumbs. Add onion balls in your air fryer's cooking basket and cook for 15 minutes. Serve and enjoy!

Nutrition Info: Calories: 162 Cal Total Fat: 12.1 g Saturated Fat: 0 g Cholesterol: 25 mg Sodium: 324 mg Total Carbs: 7.3 g Fiber: 0 g Sugar: 0 g Protein: 6 g

156.Breaded Shrimp With Lemon

Servings: 3
Cooking Time: 14 Minutes
Ingredients:
- ½ cup plain flour
- 2 egg whites
- 1 cup breadcrumbs
- 1 pound large shrimp, peeled and deveined
- Salt and ground black pepper, as required
- ¼ teaspoon lemon zest
- ¼ teaspoon cayenne pepper
- ¼ teaspoon red pepper flakes, crushed
- 2 tablespoons vegetable oil

Directions:
1. Preheat the Air fryer to 400 degree F and grease an Air fryer basket.
2. Mix flour, salt, and black pepper in a shallow bowl.
3. Whisk the egg whites in a second bowl and mix the breadcrumbs, lime zest and spices in a third bowl.
4. Coat each shrimp with the flour, dip into egg whites and finally, dredge in the breadcrumbs.
5. Drizzle the shrimp evenly with olive oil and arrange half of the coated shrimps into the Air fryer basket.
6. Cook for about 7 minutes and dish out the coated shrimps onto serving plates.
7. Repeat with the remaining mixture and serve hot.
Nutrition Info: Calories: 432, Fat: 11.3g, Carbohydrates: 44.8g, Sugar: 2.5g, Protein: 37.7g, Sodium: 526mg

157.Red Hot Chili Fish Curry

Servings: 4
Cooking Time: 20 Minutes
Ingredients:
- 2 tablespoons sunflower oil
- 1 pound fish, chopped
- 2 red chilies, chopped
- 1 tablespoon coriander powder
- 1 teaspoon red curry paste
- 1 cup coconut milk
- Salt and white pepper, to taste
- 1/2 teaspoon fenugreek seeds
- 1 shallot, minced
- 1 garlic clove, minced
- 1 ripe tomato, pureed

Directions:
1.   Preheat your Air Fryer to 380 degrees F; brush the cooking basket with 1 tablespoon of sunflower oil.
2.   Cook your fish for 10 minutes on both sides. Transfer to the baking pan that is previously greased with the remaining tablespoon of sunflower oil.
3.   Add the remaining ingredients and reduce the heat to 350 degrees F. Continue to cook an additional 10 to 12 minutes or until everything is heated through. Enjoy!
Nutrition Info: 298 Calories; 18g Fat; 4g Carbs; 23g Protein; 7g Sugars; 7g Fiber

158.Steak With Cascabel-garlic Sauce

Servings: 4
Cooking Time: 20 Minutes
Ingredients:
- 2 teaspoons brown mustard
- 2 tablespoons mayonnaise
- 1 ½ pounds beef flank steak, trimmed and cubed
- 2 teaspoons minced cascabel
- ½ cup scallions, finely chopped
- 1/3 cup Crème fraîche
- 2 teaspoons cumin seeds
- 3 cloves garlic, pressed
- Pink peppercorns to taste, freshly cracked
- 1 teaspoon fine table salt
- 1/3 teaspoon black pepper, preferably freshly ground

Directions:
1.   Firstly, fry the cumin seeds just about 1 minute or until they pop.
2.   After that, season your beef flank steak with fine table salt, black pepper and the fried cumin seeds; arrange the seasoned beef cubes on the bottom of your baking dish that fits in the air fryer.
3.   Throw in the minced cascabel, garlic, and scallions; air-fry approximately 8 minutes at 390 degrees F.
4.   Once the beef cubes start to tender, add your favorite mayo, Crème fraîche, freshly cracked pink peppercorns and mustard; air-fry 7 minutes longer. Serve over hot wild rice.
Nutrition Info: 329 Calories; 16g Fat; 8g Carbs; 37g Protein; 9g Sugars; 6g Fiber

159.Grilled Chicken Tikka Masala

Servings: 4
Cooking Time: 20 Minutes
Ingredients:
- 1 tsp. Tikka Masala 1 tsp. fine sea salt
- 2 heaping tsps. whole grain mustard
- 2 tsps. coriander, ground 2 tablespoon olive oil

- 2 large-sized chicken breasts, skinless and halved lengthwise
- 2 tsp.s onion powder
- 1½ tablespoons cider vinegar Basmati rice, steamed
- 1/3 tsp. red pepper flakes, crushed

Directions:
1.   Preheat the air fryer to 335 °For 4 minutes.
2.   Toss your chicken together with the other ingredients, minus basmati rice. Let it stand at least 3 hours.
3.   Cook for 25 minutes in your air fryer; check for doneness because the time depending on the size of the piece of chicken.
4.   Serve immediately over warm basmati rice. Enjoy!
Nutrition Info: 319 Calories; 20.1g Fat; 1.9g Carbs; 30.5g Protein; 0.1g Sugars

160.Venetian Liver

Servings: 6
Cooking Time: 15-30;
Ingredients:
- 500g veal liver
- 2 white onions
- 100g of water
- 2 tbsp vinegar
- Salt and pepper to taste

Directions:
1.   Chop the onion and put it inside the pan with the water. Set the air fryer to 1800C and cook for 20 minutes.
2.   Add the liver cut into small pieces and vinegar, close the lid, and cook for an additional 10 minutes.
3.   Add salt and pepper.
Nutrition Info: Calories 131, Fat 14.19 g, Carbohydrates 16.40 g, Sugars 5.15 g, Protein 25.39 g, Cholesterol 350.41 mg

161.Ham Rolls

Servings: 4
Cooking Time: 15 Minutes
Ingredients:
- 12-ounce refrigerated pizza crust, rolled into ¼ inch thickness
- 1/3 pound cooked ham, sliced
- ¾ cup Mozzarella cheese, shredded
- 3 cups Colby cheese, shredded
- 3-ounce roasted red bell peppers
- 1 tablespoon olive oil

Directions:
1.   Preheat the Air fryer to 360 degree F and grease an Air fryer basket.

2. Arrange the ham, cheeses and roasted peppers over one side of dough and fold to seal.
3. Brush the dough evenly with olive oil and cook for about 15 minutes, flipping twice in between.
4. Dish out in a platter and serve warm.
Nutrition Info: Calories: 594, Fat: 35.8g, Carbohydrates: 35.4g, Sugar: 2.8g, Protein: 33g, Sodium: 1545mg

162. Salmon With Crisped Topped Crumbs

Servings: 2
Cooking Time: 15 Minutes
Ingredients:
- 1-1/2 cups soft bread crumbs
- 2 tablespoons minced fresh parsley
- 1 tablespoon minced fresh thyme or 1 teaspoon dried thyme
- 2 garlic cloves, minced
- 1 teaspoon grated lemon zest
- 1/2 teaspoon salt
- 1/4 teaspoon lemon-pepper seasoning
- 1/4 teaspoon paprika
- 1 tablespoon butter, melted
- 2 salmon fillets (6 ounces each)

Directions:
1. In a medium bowl mix well bread crumbs, fresh parsley thyme, garlic, lemon zest, salt, lemon-pepper seasoning, and paprika.
2. Place the instant pot air fryer lid on, lightly grease baking pan of the instant pot with cooking spray. Add salmon fillet with skin side down. Evenly sprinkle crumbs on tops of salmon and place the baking pan in the instant pot.
3. Close the air fryer lid and cook at 390F for 10 minutes.
4. Let it rest for 5 minutes.
5. Serve and enjoy.
Nutrition Info: Calories: 331; Carbs: 9.0g; Protein: 31.0g; Fat: 19.0g

163. Hot Pork Skewers

Servings: 3 To 4
Cooking Time: 1 Hour 20 Minutes
Ingredients:
- 1 lb pork steak, cut in cubes
- ¼ cup soy sauce
- 2 tsp smoked paprika
- 1 tsp powdered chili
- 1 tsp garlic salt
- 1 tsp red chili flakes
- 1 tbsp white wine vinegar
- 3 tbsp steak sauce
- Skewing:

- 1 green pepper, cut in cubes
- 1 red pepper, cut in cubes
- 1 yellow squash, seeded and cut in cubes
- 1 green squash, seeded and cut in cubes
- Salt and black pepper to taste to season

Directions:
1. In a mixing bowl, add the pork cubes, soy sauce, smoked paprika, powdered chili, garlic salt, red chili flakes, white wine vinegar, and steak sauce. Mix them using a ladle. Refrigerate to marinate them for 1 hour.
2. After one hour, remove the marinated pork from the fridge and preheat the Air Fryer to 370 F.
3. On each skewer, stick the pork cubes and vegetables in the order that you prefer. Have fun doing this. Once the pork cubes and vegetables are finished, arrange the skewers in the fryer basket and grill them for 8 minutes. You can do them in batches. Once ready, remove them onto the serving platter and serve with salad.
Nutrition Info: 456 Calories; 37g Fat; 1g Carbs; 21g Protein; 5g Sugars; 6g Fiber

164. One-pan Shrimp And Chorizo Mix Grill

Servings: 4
Cooking Time: 15 Minutes
Ingredients:
- 1 ½ pounds large shrimps, peeled and deveined
- Salt and pepper to taste
- 6 links fresh chorizo sausage
- 2 bunches asparagus spears, trimmed
- Lime wedges

Directions:
1. Place the instant pot air fryer lid on and preheat the instant pot at 390 degrees F.
2. Place the grill pan accessory in the instant pot.
3. Season the shrimps with salt and pepper to taste. Set aside.
4. Place the chorizo on the grill pan and the sausage.
5. Place the asparagus on top.
6. Close the air fryer lid and grill for 15 minutes.
7. Serve with lime wedges.
Nutrition Info: Calories:124 ; Carbs: 9.4g; Protein: 8.2g; Fat: 7.1g

165. Couscous Stuffed Tomatoes

Servings: 4
Cooking Time: 25 Minutes
Ingredients:
- 4 tomatoes, tops and seeds removed
- 1 parsnip, peeled and finely chopped
- 1 cup mushrooms, chopped
- 1½ cups couscous

- 1 teaspoon olive oil
- 1 garlic clove, minced
- 1 tablespoon mirin sauce

Directions:
1. Preheat the Air fryer to 355 degree F and grease an Air fryer basket.
2. Heat olive oil in a skillet on low heat and add parsnips, mushrooms and garlic.
3. Cook for about 5 minutes and stir in the mirin sauce and couscous.
4. Stuff the couscous mixture into the tomatoes and arrange into the Air fryer basket.
5. Cook for about 20 minutes and dish out to serve warm.

Nutrition Info: Calories: 361, Fat: 2g, Carbohydrates: 75.5g, Sugar: 5.1g, Protein: 10.4g, Sodium: 37mg

166.Garlic Parmesan Shrimp

Servings: 2
Cooking Time: 10 Minutes
Ingredients:
- 1 pound shrimp, deveined and peeled
- ½ cup parmesan cheese, grated
- ¼ cup cilantro, diced
- 1 tablespoon olive oil
- 1 teaspoon salt
- 1 teaspoon fresh cracked pepper
- 1 tablespoon lemon juice
- 6 garlic cloves, diced

Directions:
1. Preheat the Air fryer to 350 degree F and grease an Air fryer basket.
2. Drizzle shrimp with olive oil and lemon juice and season with garlic, salt and cracked pepper.
3. Cover the bowl with plastic wrap and refrigerate for about 3 hours.
4. Stir in the parmesan cheese and cilantro to the bowl and transfer to the Air fryer basket.
5. Cook for about 10 minutes and serve immediately.

Nutrition Info: Calories: 602, Fat: 23.9g, Carbohydrates: 46.5g, Sugar: 2.9g, Protein: 11.3g, Sodium: 886mg

167.Cocktail Franks In Blanket

Servings: 4
Cooking Time: 20 Minutes
Ingredients:
- 12 oz cocktail franks
- 8 oz can crescent rolls

Directions:
1. Use a paper towel to pat the cocktail franks to drain completely. Cut the dough in 1 by 5-inch rectangles using a knife. Gently roll the franks in the strips, making sure the ends are visible place in freezer for 5 minutes.
2. Preheat the fryer to 330 f. Take the franks out of the freezer and place them in the air fryer's basket and cook for 6-8 minutes. Increase the temperature to 390 f. Cook for another 3 minutes until a fine golden texture appears.

Nutrition Info: Calories: 60 Cal Total Fat: 4.8 g Saturated Fat: 1.6 g Cholesterol: 2 mg Sodium: 136 mg Total Carbs: 2.4 g Fiber: 0.2 g Sugar: 0.1 g Protein: 1.6 g

168.Pork Belly With Honey

Servings: 8
Cooking Time: 35 Minutes
Ingredients:
- 2 pounds pork belly
- ½ tsp pepper
- 1 tbsp olive oil
- 1 tbsp salt
- 3 tbsp honey

Directions:
1. Preheat your air fryer to 400 f. Season the pork belly with salt and pepper. Grease the basket with oil. Add seasoned meat and cook for 15 minutes. Add honey and cook for 10 minutes more. Serve with green salad.

Nutrition Info: Calories: 274 Cal Total Fat: 18 g Saturated Fat: 0 g Cholesterol: 0 mg Sodium: 0 mg Total Carbs: 8 g Fiber: 0 g Sugar: 0 g Protein: 18 g

169.Fragrant Pork Tenderloin

Servings: 3
Cooking Time: 15 Minutes
Ingredients:
- ½ teaspoon saffron
- 1 teaspoon sage
- ½ teaspoon ground cinnamon
- 1 teaspoon garlic powder
- 1 teaspoon onion powder
- 1-pound pork tenderloin
- 3 tablespoon butter
- 1 garlic clove, crushed
- 1 tablespoon apple cider vinegar

Directions:
1. Combine the saffron, sage, ground cinnamon, garlic powder, and onion powder together in the shallow bowl.
2. Then shake the spices gently to make them homogenous.
3. After this, coat the pork tenderloin in the spice mixture.

4. Rub the pork tenderloin with the crushed garlic and sprinkle the meat with the apple cider vinegar.
5. Leave the pork tenderloin for 10 minutes to marinate.
6. Meanwhile, preheat the air fryer to 320 F.
7. Put the pork tenderloin in the air fryer tray and place the butter over the meat.
8. Cook the meat for 15 minutes.
9. When the meat is cooked – let it chill briefly.
10. Slice the pork tenderloin and serve it.
11. Enjoy!
Nutrition Info: calories 328, fat 16.9, fiber 0.5, carbs 2.2, protein 40

170.Lobster Lasagna Maine Style

Servings: 6
Cooking Time: 50 Minutes
Ingredients:
- 1/2 (15 ounces) container ricotta cheese
- 1 egg
- 1 cup shredded Cheddar cheese
- 1/2 cup shredded mozzarella cheese
- 1/2 cup grated Parmesan cheese
- 1/2 medium onion, minced
- 1-1/2 teaspoons minced garlic
- 1 tablespoon chopped fresh parsley
- 1/2 teaspoon freshly ground black pepper
- 1 (16 ounces) jar Alfredo pasta sauce
- 8 no-boil lasagna noodles
- 1 pound cooked and cubed lobster meat
- 5-ounce package baby spinach leaves

Directions:
1. Mix well half of Parmesan, half of the mozzarella, half of cheddar, egg, and ricotta cheese in a medium bowl. Stir in pepper, parsley, garlic, and onion.
2. Place the instant pot air fryer lid on, lightly grease baking pan of the instant pot with cooking spray.
3. On the bottom of the pan, spread ½ of the Alfredo sauce, top with a single layer of lasagna noodles. Followed by 1/3 of lobster meat, 1/3 of ricotta cheese mixture, 1/3 of spinach. Repeat layering process until all ingredients are used up.
4. Sprinkle remaining cheese on top. Shake pan to settle lasagna and burst bubbles. Cover pan with foil and place the baking pan in the instant pot.
5. Close the air fryer lid and cook at 360F for 30 minutes
6. Remove foil and cook for 10 minutes at 390F until tops are lightly browned.
7. Let it stand for 10 minutes.
8. Serve and enjoy.
Nutrition Info: Calories: 558; Carbs: 20.4g; Protein: 36.8g; Fat: 36.5g

171.Buttered Scallops

Servings: 2
Cooking Time: 4 Minutes
Ingredients:
- ¾ pound sea scallops, cleaned and patted very dry
- 1 tablespoon butter, melted
- ½ tablespoon fresh thyme, minced
- Salt and black pepper, as required

Directions:
1. Preheat the Air fryer to 390 degree F and grease an Air fryer basket.
2. Mix scallops, butter, thyme, salt, and black pepper in a bowl.
3. Arrange scallops in the Air fryer basket and cook for about 4 minutes.
4. Dish out the scallops in a platter and serve hot.
Nutrition Info: Calories: 202, Fat: 7.1g, Carbohydrates: 4.4g, Sugar: 0g, Protein: 28.7g, Sodium: 393mg

SNACKS AND DESSERTS RECIPES

172.Moist Pound Cake

Servings: 10
Cooking Time: 55 Minutes
Ingredients:
- 4 eggs
- 1 cup almond flour
- 1/2 cup sour cream
- 1 tsp vanilla
- 1 cup monk fruit sweetener
- 1/4 cup cream cheese
- 1/4 cup butter
- 1 tsp baking powder
- 1 tbsp coconut flour

Directions:
1. Fit the oven with the rack in position
2. In a large bowl, mix together almond flour, baking powder, and coconut flour.
3. In a separate bowl, add cream cheese and butter and microwave for 30 seconds. Stir well and microwave for 30 seconds more.
4. Stir in sour cream, vanilla, and sweetener. Stir well.
5. Pour cream cheese mixture into the almond flour mixture and stir until just combined.
6. Add eggs in batter one by one and stir until well combined.
7. Pour batter into the prepared grease cake pan.
8. Set to bake at 350 F for 60 minutes. After 5 minutes place the cake pan in the preheated oven.
9. Slice and serve.
Nutrition Info: Calories 210 Fat 17 g Carbohydrates 8 g Sugar 5 g Protein 3 g Cholesterol 89 mg

173.Vanilla Peanut Butter Cake

Servings: 8
Cooking Time: 30 Minutes
Ingredients:
- 1 1/2 cups all-purpose flour
- 1/3 cup vegetable oil
- 1 tsp baking soda
- 1/2 cup peanut butter powder
- 1 tsp vanilla
- 1 tbsp apple cider vinegar
- 1 cup of water
- 1 cup of sugar
- 1/2 tsp salt

Directions:
1. Fit the oven with the rack in position
2. In a large mixing bowl, mix together flour, baking soda, peanut butter powder, sugar, and salt.
3. In a small bowl, whisk together oil, vanilla, vinegar, and water.
4. Pour oil mixture into the flour mixture and stir until well combined.
5. Pour batter into the greased cake pan.
6. Set to bake at 350 F for 35 minutes. After 5 minutes place the cake pan in the preheated oven.
7. Slice and serve.
Nutrition Info: Calories 264 Fat 1.8 g Carbohydrates 43.2 g Sugar 25.3 g Protein 2.6 g Cholesterol 0 mg

174.Plum Cream(2)

Servings: 4
Cooking Time: 15 Minutes
Ingredients:
- 1 lb. plums, pitted and chopped.
- 1 ½ cups heavy cream
- ¼ cup swerve
- 1 tbsp. lemon juice

Directions:
1. Take a bowl and mix all the ingredients and whisk really well.
2. Divide this into 4 ramekins, put them in the air fryer and cook at 340°F for 20 minutes. Serve cold
Nutrition Info: Calories: 171; Fat: 4g; Fiber: 2g; Carbs: 4g; Protein: 4g

175.Healthy Sesame Bars

Servings: 16
Cooking Time: 15 Minutes
Ingredients:
- 1 1/4 cups sesame seeds
- 1/4 cup applesauce
- 3/4 cup coconut butter
- 10 drops liquid stevia
- 1/2 tsp vanilla
- Pinch of salt

Directions:
1. Fit the oven with the rack in position
2. In a large bowl, add applesauce, coconut butter, vanilla, liquid stevia, and sea salt and stir until well combined.
3. Add sesame seeds and stir to coat.
4. Pour mixture into a greased baking dish.
5. Set to bake at 350 F for 20 minutes. After 5 minutes place the baking dish in the preheated oven.
6. Cut into pieces and serve.
Nutrition Info: Calories 136 Fat 12.4 g Carbohydrates 5.7 g Sugar 1.2 g Protein 2.8 g Cholesterol 0 mg

176.Tofu Steaks

Servings: 4

Cooking Time: 35 Minutes
Ingredients:
- 1 package tofu, press and remove excess liquid
- 2 tbsp lemon zest
- 3 garlic cloves, minced
- 1/4 cup olive oil
- 1/4 tsp dried thyme
- 1/4 cup lemon juice
- Pepper
- Salt

Directions:
1. Fit the oven with the rack in position 2.
2. Cut tofu into eight pieces.
3. In a bowl, mix together olive oil, thyme, lemon juice, lemon zest, garlic, pepper, and salt.
4. Add tofu into the bowl and coat well and place it in the refrigerator overnight.
5. Place marinated tofu in an air fryer basket then places an air fryer basket in the baking pan.
6. Place a baking pan on the oven rack. Set to air fry at 350 F for 35 minutes.
7. Serve and enjoy.

Nutrition Info: Calories 139 Fat 14.1 g Carbohydrates 2.3 g Sugar 0.7 g Protein 2.9 g Cholesterol 0 mg

177.Chocolate Cake

Servings: 8
Cooking Time: 30 Minutes
Ingredients:
- 1/2 cup warm water
- 2 3/4 cups flour
- 1 cup buttermilk
- 1 cup shortening
- 1 cup sugar, granulated
- 1 cup brown sugar
- 2 large eggs
- 1/2 cup cocoa powder
- 1 tsp baking soda

Directions:
1. Fit the oven with the rack in position
2. In a large mixing bowl, beat together brown sugar, granulated sugar, and shortening until creamy.
3. Add eggs, cocoa powder, flour, and buttermilk mix well until combine.
4. Dissolve soda in warm water and stir into batter.
5. Pour batter into the greased baking dish.
6. Set to bake at 350 F for 35 minutes. After 5 minutes place the baking dish in the preheated oven.
7. Slices and serve.

Nutrition Info: Calories 588 Fat 28.3 g Carbohydrates 80.1 g Sugar 44.4 g Protein 8 g Cholesterol 48 mg

178.Mini Pancakes

Ingredients:
- 2 tsp. dried parsley
- Salt and Pepper to taste
- 3 tbsp. Butter
- 1 ½ cups almond flour
- 3 eggs
- 2 tsp. dried basil

Directions:
1. Preheat the air fryer to 250 Fahrenheit.
2. In a small bowl, mix the ingredients together. Ensure that the mixture is smooth and well balanced.
3. Take a pancake mold and grease it with butter. Add the batter to the mold and place it in the air fryer basket. Cook till both the sides of the pancake have browned on both sides and serve with maple syrup.

179.Buttered Dinner Rolls

Servings: 12
Cooking Time: 30 Minutes
Ingredients:
- 1 cup milk
- 3 cups plain flour
- 7½ tablespoons unsalted butter
- 1 tablespoon coconut oil
- 1 tablespoon olive oil
- 1 teaspoon yeast
- Salt and black pepper, to taste

Directions:
1. Preheat the Air fryer to 360 degree F and grease an Air fryer basket.
2. Put olive oil, milk and coconut oil in a pan and cook for about 3 minutes.
3. Remove from the heat and mix well.
4. Mix together plain flour, yeast, butter, salt and black pepper in a large bowl.
5. Knead well for about 5 minutes until a dough is formed.
6. Cover the dough with a damp cloth and keep aside for about 5 minutes in a warm place.
7. Knead the dough for about 5 minutes again with your hands.
8. Cover the dough with a damp cloth and keep aside for about 30 minutes in a warm place.
9. Divide the dough into 12 equal pieces and roll each into a ball.
10. Arrange 6 balls into the Air fryer basket in a single layer and cook for about 15 minutes.
11. Repeat with the remaining balls and serve warm.

Nutrition Info: Calories: 208, Fat: 10.3g, Carbohydrates: 25g, Sugar: 1g, Protein: 4.1g, Sodium: 73mg

180.Beefy Mini Pies

Ingredients:
- 1 cup shredded Colby cheese
- 2 eggs
- ½ cup half-and-half
- ½ teaspoon dried dill weed
- 1 (10-ounce) package refrigerated flaky dinner rolls
- ½ pound ground beef
- 1 small onion, chopped
- 2 cloves garlic, minced

Directions:
1. Preheat oven to 350ºF. Remove rolls from package and divide each roll into 3 rounds. Place each round into a 3-inch muffin cup; press firmly onto bottom and up sides.
2. In a heavy skillet, cook ground beef with onion and garlic until beef is done. Drain well. Place 1 tablespoon beef mixture into each dough-lined muffin cup. Sprinkle cheese over beef mixture. In a small bowl, beat together eggs, half-and-half, and dill weed. Spoon this mixture over beef in muffin cups, making sure not to overfill cups.
3. Bake at 350ºF for 10 to 13 minutes or until filling is puffed and set. Flash freeze in single layer on baking sheet. When frozen solid, wrap, label, and freeze.
4. To thaw and reheat: Thaw pies in single layer in refrigerator overnight. Bake at 350ºF for 7 to 9 minutes or until hot.

181.Italian Pork Skewers

Ingredients:
- ¼ cup finely minced onion
- 1 teaspoon dried Italian seasoning
- ½ teaspoon salt
- teaspoon pepper
- 2 pounds pork tenderloin
- ¼ cup balsamic vinegar
- ¼ cup olive oil

Directions:
1. Trim excess fat from tenderloin. Cut pork, on a slant, into ¼-inch-thick slices, each about 4 inches long. In large bowl, combine remaining ingredients and mix well with wire whisk. Add tenderloin slices and mix gently to coat. Cover and refrigerate for 2 to 3 hours. Meanwhile, soak 8-inch wooden skewers in cold water.
2. Remove pork from marinade and thread onto soaked skewers. Flash freeze on baking sheet in single layer. When frozen solid, pack skewers in rigid containers, with layers separated by waxed paper. Label skewers and freeze.

3. To thaw and reheat: Thaw overnight in refrigerator. Cook skewers 4 to 6 inches from medium coals on grill, or broil 4 to 6 inches from heat source, for about 4 to 6 minutes or until cooked (160ºF on an instant-read thermometer), turning once.

182.Vanilla Rum Cookies With Walnuts

Servings: 6
Cooking Time: 15 Minutes
Ingredients:
- 1/2 cup almond flour
- 1/2 cup coconut flour
- 1/2 teaspoon baking powder
- 1/4 teaspoon fine sea salt
- 1 stick butter, unsalted and softened
- 1/2 cup swerve
- 1 egg
- 1/2 teaspoon vanilla
- 1 teaspoon butter rum flavoring
- 3 ounces walnuts, finely chopped

Directions:
1. Begin by preheating the Air Fryer to 360 degrees F.
2. In a mixing dish, thoroughly combine the flour with baking powder and salt.
3. Beat the butter and swerve with a hand mixer until pale and fluffy; add the whisked egg, vanilla, and butter rum flavoring; mix again to combine well. Now, stir in the dry ingredients.
4. Fold in the chopped walnuts and mix to combine. Divide the mixture into small balls; flatten each ball with a fork and transfer them to a foil-lined baking pan.
5. Bake in the preheated Air Fryer for 14 minutes. Work in a few batches and transfer to wire racks to cool completely.
Nutrition Info: 314 Calories; 32g Fat; 7g Carbs; 2g Protein; 2g Sugars; 5g Fiber

183.Avocado Bites

Servings: 4
Cooking Time: 15 Minutes
Ingredients:
- 4 avocados, peeled, pitted and cut into wedges
- 1 ½ cups almond meal
- 1 egg; whisked
- A pinch of salt and black pepper
- Cooking spray

Directions:
1. Put the egg in a bowl and the almond meal in another.

2. Season avocado wedges with salt and pepper, coat them in egg and then in meal almond
3. Arrange the avocado bites in your air fryer's basket, grease them with cooking spray and cook at 400°F for 8 minutes. Serve as a snack right away
Nutrition Info: Calories: 200; Fat: 12g; Fiber: 3g; Carbs: 5g; Protein: 16g

184.Tangy Fried Pickle Spears

Servings: 6
Cooking Time: 15 Minutes
Ingredients:
- 2 jars sweet and sour pickle spears, patted dry
- 2 medium-sized eggs
- $^1/_3$ cup milk
- 1 teaspoon garlic powder
- 1 teaspoon sea salt
- ½ teaspoon shallot powder
- $^1/_3$ teaspoon chili powder
- $^1/_3$ cup all-purpose flour
- Cooking spray

Directions:
1. Spritz the air fryer basket with cooking spray.
2. In a bowl, beat together the eggs with milk. In another bowl, combine garlic powder, sea salt, shallot powder, chili powder and all-purpose flour until well blended.
3. One by one, roll the pickle spears in the powder mixture, then dredge them in the egg mixture. Dip them in the powder mixture a second time for additional coating.
4. Place the coated pickles in the basket.
5. Put the air fryer basket on the baking pan and slide into Rack Position 2, select Air Fry, set temperature to 385ºF (196ºC), and set time to 15 minutes.
6. Stir the pickles halfway through the cooking time.
7. When cooking is complete, they should be golden and crispy. Transfer to a plate and let cool for 5 minutes before serving.

185.Chocolate Coffee Cake

Servings: 8
Cooking Time: 15 Minutes
Ingredients:
- 1 ½ cups almond flour
- 1/2 cup coconut meal
- 2/3 cup swerve
- 1 teaspoon baking powder
- 1/4 teaspoon salt
- 1 stick butter, melted
- 1/2 cup hot strongly brewed coffee

- 1/2 teaspoon vanilla
- 1 egg
- Topping:
- 1/4 cup coconut flour
- 1/2 cup confectioner's swerve
- 1/2 teaspoon ground cardamom
- 1 teaspoon ground cinnamon
- 3 tablespoons coconut oil

Directions:
1. Mix all dry ingredients for your cake; then, mix in the wet ingredients. Mix until everything is well incorporated.
2. Spritz a baking pan with cooking spray. Scrape the batter into the baking pan.
3. Then, make the topping by mixing all ingredients. Place on top of the cake.Smooth the top with a spatula.
4. Bake at 330 degrees F for 30 minutes or until the top of the cake springs back when gently pressed with your fingers. Serve with your favorite hot beverage.
Nutrition Info: 285 Calories; 21g Fat; 6g Carbs; 8g Protein; 3g Sugars; 1g Fiber

186.Vanilla Lemon Cupcakes

Servings: 6
Cooking Time: 15 Minutes
Ingredients:
- 1 egg
- 1/2 cup milk
- 2 tbsp canola oil
- 1/4 tsp baking soda
- 3/4 tsp baking powder
- 1 tsp lemon zest, grated
- 1/2 cup sugar
- 1 cup flour
- 1/2 tsp vanilla
- 1/2 tsp salt

Directions:
1. Fit the oven with the rack in position
2. Line 12-cups muffin tin with cupcake liners and set aside.
3. In a bowl, whisk egg, vanilla, milk, oil, and sugar until creamy.
4. Add remaining ingredients and stir until just combined.
5. Pour batter into the prepared muffin tin.
6. Set to bake at 350 F for 20 minutes. After 5 minutes place muffin tin in the preheated oven.
7. Serve and enjoy.
Nutrition Info: Calories 200 Fat 6 g Carbohydrates 35 g Sugar 17 g Protein 3 g Cholesterol 30 mg

187.Mozzarella And Tomato Salad

Servings: 6
Cooking Time: 15 Minutes
Ingredients:
- 1 lb. tomatoes; sliced
- 1 cup mozzarella; shredded
- 1 tbsp. ginger; grated
- 1 tbsp. balsamic vinegar
- 1 tsp. sweet paprika
- 1 tsp. chili powder
- ½ tsp. coriander, ground

Directions:
1. In a pan that fits your air fryer, mix all the ingredients except the mozzarella, toss, introduce the pan in the air fryer and cook at 360°F for 12 minutes
2. Divide into bowls and serve cold as an appetizer with the mozzarella sprinkled all over.

Nutrition Info: Calories: 185; Fat: 8g; Fiber: 2g; Carbs: 4g; Protein: 8g

188.Crispy Coated Peaches

Servings: 1
Cooking Time: 10 Minutes
Ingredients:
- Nonstick cooking spray
- ¼ cup panko bread crumbs
- 1 tsp sugar
- ¼ tsp cinnamon
- 1/8 tsp salt
- 2 egg whites
- ¼ tsp vanilla
- 1 peach, pitted and cut in ½-inch thick slices

Directions:
1. Place baking pan in position 2. Lightly spray fryer basket with cooking spray.
2. In a medium bowl, combine bread crumbs, sugar, cinnamon, and salt.
3. In a separate medium bowl, whisk together egg whites and vanilla.
4. Add peaches to egg mixture and stir to coat. One at a time, shake off excess egg and coat with crumb mixture. Place in basket in a single layer.
5. Place basket on the baking pan and set oven to air fry on 390°F for 8 minutes. Cook until golden brown and crispy. Serve immediately topped with yogurt or whip cream.

Nutrition Info: Calories 222, Total Fat 2g, Saturated Fat 0g, Total Carbs 39g, Net Carbs 35g, Protein 12g, Sugar 19g, Fiber 4g, Sodium 617mg, Potassium 450mg, Phosphorus 85mg

189.Homemade Doughnuts

Servings: 4

Cooking Time: 25 Minutes
Ingredients:
- 8 oz self-rising flour
- 1 tsp baking powder
- ½ cup milk
- 2 ½ tbsp butter
- 1 egg
- 2 oz brown sugar

Directions:
1. Preheat on Bake function to 350 F. Beat the butter with the sugar until smooth. Whisk in the egg and milk. In a bowl, combine flour with baking powder. Fold in the butter mixture.
2. Form donut shapes and cut off the center with cookie cutters. Arrange on a lined baking sheet and cook in for 15 minutes. Serve with whipped cream or icing.

190.Strawberry Pudding

Ingredients:
- 3 tbsp. powdered sugar
- 3 tbsp. unsalted butter
- 1 cup strawberry slices
- 1 cup strawberry juice
- 2 cups milk
- 2 tbsp. custard powder

Directions:
1. Boil the milk and the sugar in a pan and add the custard powder followed by the strawberry juice and stir till you get a thick mixture.
2. Preheat the fryer to 300 Fahrenheit for five minutes. Place the dish in the basket and reduce the temperature to 250 Fahrenheit. Cook for ten minutes and set aside to cool. Garnish with strawberry.

191.Berry Crumble With Lemon

Servings: 6
Cooking Time: 30 Minutes
Ingredients:
- 12 oz fresh strawberries
- 7 oz fresh raspberries
- 5 oz fresh blueberries
- 5 tbsp cold butter
- 2 tbsp lemon juice
- 1 cup flour
- ½ cup sugar
- 1 tbsp water
- A pinch of salt

Directions:
1. Preheat Breville on Bake function to 360 F. Gently mash the berries, but make sure there are chunks left. Mix with the lemon juice and 2 tbsp of sugar. Place the berry mixture at the bottom of a

greased cake pan. Combine the flour with salt and sugar in a bowl. Mix well.
2.   Add the water and rub the butter with your fingers until the mixture becomes crumbled. Pour the batter over the berries. Press Start and cook for 20 minutes. Serve chilled.

192.Easy Spanish Churros

Servings: 4
Cooking Time: 15 Minutes
Ingredients:
- 3/4 cup water
- 1 tablespoon swerve
- 1/4 teaspoon sea salt
- 1/4 teaspoon grated nutmeg
- 1/4 teaspoon ground cloves
- 6 tablespoons butter
- 3/4 cup almond flour
- 2 eggs

Directions:
1.   To make the dough, boil the water in a pan over medium-high heat; now, add the swerve, salt, nutmeg, and cloves; cook until dissolved.
2.   Add the butter and turn the heat to low. Gradually stir in the almond flour, whisking continuously, until the mixture forms a ball.
3.   Remove from the heat; fold in the eggs one at a time, stirring to combine well.
4.   Pour the mixture into a piping bag with a large star tip. Squeeze 4-inch strips of dough into the greased Air Fryer pan.
5.   Cook at 410 degrees F for 6 minutes, working in batches.
Nutrition Info: 321 Calories; 31g Fat; 4g Carbs; 4g Protein; 1g Sugars; 3g Fiber

193.Easy Blackberry Cobbler

Servings: 6
Cooking Time: 20 To 25 Minutes
Ingredients:
- 3 cups fresh or frozen blackberries
- 1¾ cups sugar, divided
- 1 teaspoon vanilla extract
- 8 tablespoons (1 stick) butter, melted
- 1 cup self-rising flour
- Cooking spray

Directions:
1.   Spritz the baking pan with cooking spray.
2.   Mix the blackberries, 1 cup of sugar, and vanilla in a medium bowl and stir to combine.
3.   Stir together the melted butter, remaining sugar, and flour in a separate medium bowl.

4.   Spread the blackberry mixture evenly in the prepared pan and top with the butter mixture.
5.   Slide the baking pan into Rack Position 1, select Convection Bake, set temperature to 350ºF (180ºC), and set time to 25 minutes.
6.   After about 20 minutes, check if the cobbler has a golden crust and you can't see any batter bubbling while it cooks. If needed, bake for another 5 minutes.
7.   Remove from the oven and place on a wire rack to cool to room temperature. Serve immediately.

194.Fudge Brownies

Servings: 8
Cooking Time: 20 Minutes
Ingredients:
- 1 cup sugar
- ½ cup butter, melted
- ½ cup flour
- 1/3 cup cocoa powder
- 1 teaspoon baking powder
- 2 eggs
- 1 teaspoon vanilla extract

Directions:
1.   Grease a baking pan.
2.   In a large bowl, add the sugar, and butter and whisk until light and fluffy.
3.   Add the remaining ingredients and mix until well combined.
4.   Place mixture into the prepared pan and with the back of spatula, smooth the top surface.
5.   Press "Power Button" of Air Fry Oven and turn the dial to select the "Air Fry" mode.
6.   Press the Time button and again turn the dial to set the cooking time to 20 minutes.
7.   Now push the Temp button and rotate the dial to set the temperature at 350 degrees F.
8.   Press "Start/Pause" button to start.
9.   When the unit beeps to show that it is preheated, open the lid.
10.   Arrange the pan in "Air Fry Basket" and insert in the oven.
11.   Place the baking pan onto a wire rack to cool completely.
12.   Cut into 8 equal-sized squares and serve.
Nutrition Info: Calories 250 Total Fat 13.2 g Saturated Fat 7.9 g Cholesterol 71 mg Sodium 99 mg Total Carbs 33.4 g Fiber 1.3 g Sugar 25.2 g Protein 3 g

195.Sweet And Sour Meatballs

Ingredients:
- ¼ cup apple cider vinegar
- 1 (10-ounce) can condensed tomato soup
- cup sugar

- 1 (8-ounce) can pineapple tidbits, undrained
- 1-pound ground beef
- 1 egg
- ½ cup grated Parmesan cheese
- ¼ cup dry bread crumbs

Directions:
1. Preheat oven to 350ºF. In medium bowl, combine ground beef, egg, cheese, and bread crumbs and mix well to blend. Form into 1-inch meatballs and place on baking sheet. Bake at 350ºF for 20 to 25 minutes or until no longer pink in center. Chill meatballs in refrigerator until thoroughly cold.
2. In a medium bowl, combine vinegar, soup, sugar, and pineapple tidbits and juice. Mix well and pour into 1-gallon-size zipper-lock freezer bag. Add meatballs, seal bag, and turn gently to mix. Label bag and freeze.
3. To thaw and reheat: Thaw overnight in refrigerator. Pour meatballs and sauce into large skillet and cook over medium heat until sauce comes to a boil. Reduce heat, cover, and simmer meatballs for 8 to 10 minutes or until thoroughly heated, stirring occasionally.

196.Sausage And Mushroom Empanadas

Servings: 4
Cooking Time: 12 Minutes
Ingredients:
- ½ pound (227 g) Kielbasa smoked sausage, chopped
- 4 chopped canned mushrooms
- 2 tablespoons chopped onion
- ½ teaspoon ground cumin
- ¼ teaspoon paprika
- Salt and black pepper, to taste
- ½ package puff pastry dough, at room temperature
- 1 egg, beaten
- Cooking spray

Directions:
1. Combine the sausage, mushrooms, onion, cumin, paprika, salt, and pepper in a bowl and stir to mix well.
2. Make the empanadas: Place the puff pastry dough on a lightly floured surface. Cut circles into the dough with a glass. Place 1 tablespoon of the sausage mixture into the center of each pastry circle. Fold each in half and pinch the edges to seal. Using a fork, crimp the edges. Brush them with the beaten egg and mist with cooking spray.
3. Spritz the air fryer basket with cooking spray. Place the empanadas in the basket.
4. Put the air fryer basket on the baking pan and slide into Rack Position 2, select Air Fry, set

temperature to 360ºF (182ºC), and set time to 12 minutes.
5. Flip the empanadas halfway through the cooking time.
6. When cooking is complete, the empanadas should be golden brown. Remove from the oven. Allow them to cool for 5 minutes and serve hot.

197.Buffalo Style Cauliflower

Ingredients:
- ¼ cup Frank's red-hot sauce
- 1 Tbsp fresh lime juice
- Chopped parsley or cilantro
- 2 Tbsp olive oil
- 1 head cauliflower
- Salt and pepper, to taste
- 2 Tbsp unsalted butter

Directions:
1. Preheat oven to 375°F.
2. Chop off tough flower part at the base of the cauliflower. Break into
3. small to medium sized florets.
4. In a microwave-safe bowl, melt butter.
5. Add hot sauce and lime juice to butter and stir.
6. Heat oven to medium-low heat.
7. Add oil and cauliflower florets. Saute until nicely browned, 4-5 minutes.
8. Pour in hot sauce mixture and stir to coat evenly.
9. Place in oven for 15-20 minutes, until cauliflower is softened.
10. Remove from oven and sprinkle with parsley or cilantro.

198.Garlic Cheese Dip

Servings: 10
Cooking Time: 15 Minutes
Ingredients:
- 1 lb. mozzarella; shredded
- 6 garlic cloves; minced
- 3 tbsp. olive oil
- 1 tbsp. thyme; chopped.
- 1 tsp. rosemary; chopped.
- A pinch of salt and black pepper

Directions:
1. In a pan that fits your air fryer, mix all the ingredients, whisk really well, introduce in the air fryer and cook at 370°F for 10 minutes.
2. Divide into bowls and serve right away.
Nutrition Info: Calories: 184; Fat: 11g; Fiber: 3g; Carbs: 5g; Protein: 7g

199.Sunflower Seeds Bread

Servings: 4
Cooking Time: 18 Minutes
Ingredients:
- 2/3 cup whole wheat flour
- 2/3 cup plain flour
- 1/3 cup sunflower seeds
- 1 cup lukewarm water
- ½ sachet instant yeast
- 1 teaspoon salt

Directions:
1. Preheat the Air fryer to 390 degree F and grease a cake pan.
2. Mix together flours, sunflower seeds, yeast and salt in a bowl.
3. Add water slowly and knead for about 5 minutes until a dough is formed.
4. Cover the dough with a plastic wrap and keep in warm place for about half an hour.
5. Arrange the dough into a cake pan and transfer into an Air fryer basket.
6. Cook for about 18 minutes and dish out to serve warm.

Nutrition Info: Calories: 156, Fat: 2.4g, Carbohydrates: 28.5g, Sugar: 0.5g, Protein: 4.6g, Sodium: 582mg

200.Spicy Chicken Wings

Servings: 6
Cooking Time: 16 Minutes
Ingredients:
- 1/2 lb chicken wings
- 2 tsp ginger powder
- 1 tsp paprika
- 1/3 cup hot sauce
- 2 tsp garlic powder
- Pepper
- Salt

Directions:
1. Fit the oven with the rack in position 2.
2. Toss chicken wings with paprika, garlic powder, pepper, ginger powder, and salt.
3. Add chicken wings to the air fryer basket then place an air fryer basket in the baking pan.
4. Place a baking pan on the oven rack. Set to air fry at 360 F for 16 minutes.
5. Serve with hot sauce.

Nutrition Info: Calories 104 Fat 2.9 g Carbohydrates 5.8 g Sugar 3.9 g Protein 11.2 g Cholesterol 34 mg

201.Date Bread

Servings: 10
Cooking Time: 20 Minutes

Ingredients:
- ¼ cup of butter
- 1½ cups of flour
- 1 teaspoon of baking powder
- ½ teaspoon of salt
- 2½ cup of dates, pitted and chopped
- 1 cup of hot water
- ½ cup of brown sugar
- 1 teaspoon of baking soda
- 1 egg

Directions:
1. Set the Instant Vortex on Air fryer to 340 degrees F for 20 minutes. Combine dates with butter and hot water in a bowl. Strain together brown sugar, flour, baking powder, baking soda, and salt in another bowl. Fold the brown sugar mixture and egg in the date's mixture. Place the mixture on the cooking tray. Insert the cooking tray in the Vortex when it displays "Add Food". Flip the sides when it displays "Turn Food". Remove from the oven when cooking time is complete. Slice into desired pieces to serve.

Nutrition Info: Calories: 269 Cal Total Fat: 5.4 g Saturated Fat: 0 g Cholesterol: 0 mg Sodium: 0 mg Total Carbs: 55.1 g Fiber: 0 g Sugar: 0 g Protein: 3.6 g

202.Cinnamon Fried Bananas

Servings: 2-3
Cooking Time: 10 Minutes
Ingredients:
- 1 C. panko breadcrumbs
- 3 tbsp. cinnamon
- ½ C. almond flour
- 3 egg whites
- 8 ripe bananas
- 3 tbsp. vegan coconut oil

Directions:
1. Preparing the Ingredients. Heat coconut oil and add breadcrumbs. Mix around 2-3 minutes until golden. Pour into bowl.
2. Peel and cut bananas in half. Roll each bananas half into flour, eggs, and crumb mixture.
3. Air Frying. Place into the air fryer oven. Cook 10 minutes at 280 degrees.
4. A great addition to a healthy banana split!

Nutrition Info: CALORIES: 219; FAT:10G; PROTEIN:3G; SUGAR:5G

203.Easy Air Fryer Tofu

Servings: 4
Cooking Time: 15 Minutes
Ingredients:

- 16 oz extra firm tofu, cut into bite-sized pieces
- 1 tbsp olive oil
- 1 garlic clove, minced

Directions:
1. Fit the oven with the rack in position 2.
2. Add tofu, garlic, and oil in a mixing bowl and toss well. Let it sit for 15 minutes.
3. Arrange tofu in the air fryer basket then place an air fryer basket in the baking pan.
4. Place a baking pan on the oven rack. Set to air fry at 370 F for 15 minutes.
5. Serve and enjoy.

Nutrition Info: Calories 111 Fat 8.2 g Carbohydrates 2.2 g Sugar 0.7 g Protein 9.3 g Cholesterol 0 mg

204.Walnut Brownies

Servings: 4
Cooking Time: 22 Minutes
Ingredients:
- ½ cup chocolate, roughly chopped
- 1/3 cup butter
- 5 tablespoons sugar
- 1 egg, beaten
- 1 teaspoon vanilla extract
- Pinch of salt
- 5 tablespoons self-rising flour
- ¼ cup walnuts, chopped

Directions:
1. In a microwave-safe bowl, add the chocolate and butter. Microwave on high heat for about 2 minutes, stirring after every 30 seconds.
2. Remove from microwave and set aside to cool.
3. In another bowl, add the sugar, egg, vanilla extract, and salt and whisk until creamy and light.
4. Add the chocolate mixture and whisk until well combined.
5. Add the flour, and walnuts and mix until well combined.
6. Line a baking pan with a greased parchment paper.
7. Place mixture evenly into the prepared pan and with the back of spatula, smooth the top surface.
8. Press "Power Button" of Air Fry Oven and turn the dial to select the "Air Fry" mode.
9. Press the Time button and again turn the dial to set the cooking time to 20 minutes.
10. Now push the Temp button and rotate the dial to set the temperature at 355 degrees F.
11. Press "Start/Pause" button to start.
12. When the unit beeps to show that it is preheated, open the lid.
13. Arrange the pan in "Air Fry Basket" and insert in the oven.
14. Place the baking pan onto a wire rack to cool completely.

15. Cut into 4 equal-sized squares and serve.
Nutrition Info: Calories 407 Total Fat 27.4g Saturated Fat 14.7 g Cholesterol 86 mg Sodium 180 mg Total Carbs 35.9 g Fiber 1.5 g Sugar 26.2 g Protein 6 g

205.Polenta Fries With Chili-lime Mayo

Servings: 4
Cooking Time: 28 Minutes
Ingredients:
- Polenta Fries:
- 2 teaspoons vegetable or olive oil
- ¼ teaspoon paprika
- 1 pound (454 g) prepared polenta, cut into 3-inch × ½-inch strips
- Salt and freshly ground black pepper, to taste
- Chili-Lime Mayo:
- ½ cup mayonnaise
- 1 teaspoon chili powder
- 1 teaspoon chopped fresh cilantro
- ¼ teaspoon ground cumin
- Juice of ½ lime
- Salt and freshly ground black pepper, to taste

Directions:
1. Mix the oil and paprika in a bowl. Add the polenta strips and toss until evenly coated. Transfer the polenta strips to the air fryer basket.
2. Put the air fryer basket on the baking pan and slide into Rack Position 2, select Air Fry, set temperature to 400ºF (205ºC), and set time to 28 minutes.
3. Stir the polenta strips halfway through the cooking time.
4. Meanwhile, whisk together all the ingredients for the chili-lime mayo in a small bowl.
5. When cooking is complete, remove the polenta fries from the oven to a plate. Season as desired with salt and pepper. Serve alongside the chili-lime mayo as a dipping sauce.

206.Honey And Orange Pancakes

Ingredients:
- 2 tsp. dried basil
- 2 tsp. dried parsley
- Salt and Pepper to taste
- 3 tbsp. Butter
- 1 orange (zested)
- 1 ½ cups almond flour
- 3 eggs
- 1 tbsp. honey

Directions:
1. Preheat the air fryer to 250 Fahrenheit.

2. In a small bowl, mix the ingredients together. Ensure that the mixture is smooth and well balanced.
3. Take a pancake mold and grease it with butter. Add the batter to the mold and place it in the air fryer basket.
4. Cook till both the sides of the pancake have browned on both sides and serve with maple syrup.

207.Blackberry Chocolate Cake

Servings: 8
Cooking Time: 22 Minutes
Ingredients:
- ½ cup butter, at room temperature
- 2 ounces (57 g) Swerve
- 4 eggs
- 1 cup almond flour
- 1 teaspoon baking soda
- $1/3$ teaspoon baking powder
- ½ cup cocoa powder
- 1 teaspoon orange zest
- $1/3$ cup fresh blackberries

Directions:
1. With an electric mixer or hand mixer, beat the butter and Swerve until creamy.
2. One at a time, mix in the eggs and beat again until fluffy.
3. Add the almond flour, baking soda, baking powder, cocoa powder, orange zest and mix well. Add the butter mixture to the almond flour mixture and stir until well blended. Fold in the blackberries.
4. Scrape the batter into the baking pan.
5. Slide the baking pan into Rack Position 1, select Convection Bake, set temperature to 335ºF (168ºC), and set time to 22 minutes.
6. When cooking is complete, a toothpick inserted into the center of the cake should come out clean.
7. Allow the cake cool on a wire rack to room temperature. Serve immediately.

208.Apple-peach Crumble With Honey

Servings: 4
Cooking Time: 11 Minutes
Ingredients:
- 1 apple, peeled and chopped
- 2 peaches, peeled, pitted, and chopped
- 2 tablespoons honey
- ½ cup quick-cooking oatmeal
- $1/3$ cup whole-wheat pastry flour
- 2 tablespoons unsalted butter, at room temperature
- 3 tablespoons packed brown sugar
- ½ teaspoon ground cinnamon

Directions:

1. Mix together the apple, peaches, and honey in the baking pan until well incorporated.
2. In a bowl, combine the oatmeal, pastry flour, butter, brown sugar, and cinnamon and stir to mix well. Spread this mixture evenly over the fruit.
3. Slide the baking pan into Rack Position 1, select Convection Bake, set temperature to 380ºF (193ºC), and set time to 11 minutes.
4. When cooking is complete, the fruit should be bubbling around the edges and the topping should be golden brown.
5. Remove from the oven and serve warm.

209.Baked Yoghurt

Ingredients:
- 1 cup blackberries
- Handful of mint leaves
- 3 tsp. sugar
- 4 tsp. water
- 2 cups condensed milk
- 2 cups yoghurt
- 2 cups fresh cream
- 1 cup fresh strawberries
- 1 cup fresh blueberries

Directions:
1. Mix the ingredients together and create a thick mixture. Transfer this into baking bowls ensuring that you do not overfill.
2. Preheat the fryer to 300 Fahrenheit for five minutes. You will need to place the bowls in the basket and cover it. Cook it for fifteen minutes. When you shake the bowls, the mixture should just shake but not break. Leave it in the refrigerator to set and then arrange the fruits, garnish and serve.

210.Choco-peanut Mug Cake

Servings: 1
Cooking Time: 20 Minutes
Ingredients:
- Softened butter, 1 tsp.
- Egg, 1.
- Peanut butter, 1 tbsp.
- Vanilla extract, ½ tsp.
- Erythritol, 2 tbsps.
- Unsweetened cocoa powder, 2 tbsps.
- Baking powder, ¼ tsp.
- Heavy cream, 1 tbsp.

Directions:
1. Preheat the air fryer for 5 minutes.
2. Combine all ingredients in a mixing bowl.
3. Pour into a greased mug.
4. Set in the air fryer basket and cook for 20 minutes at 400F

Nutrition Info: Calories: 293 Protein: 12.4g Fat: 23.3g Carbs: 8.5g

211.Air Fryer Pepperoni Chips

Servings: 6
Cooking Time: 8 Minutes
Ingredients:
- 6 oz pepperoni slices

Directions:
1. Fit the oven with the rack in position 2.
2. Place pepperoni slices in an air fryer basket then place an air fryer basket in baking pan.
3. Place a baking pan on the oven rack. Set to air fry at 360 F for 8 minutes.
4. Serve and enjoy.

Nutrition Info: Calories 51 Fat 1 g Carbohydrates 2 g Sugar 0 g Protein 9.1 g Cholesterol 0 mg

212.Banana Butter Brownie

Servings: 4
Cooking Time: 16 Minutes
Ingredients:
- 1 scoop protein powder
- 2 tbsp cocoa powder
- 1 cup bananas, overripe
- 1/2 cup almond butter, melted

Directions:
1. Fit the oven with the rack in position
2. Add all ingredients into the blender and blend until smooth.
3. Pour batter into the greased cake pan.
4. Set to bake at 325 F for 21 minutes. After 5 minutes place the cake pan in the preheated oven.
5. Serve and enjoy.

Nutrition Info: Calories 83 Fat 2 g Carbohydrates 10 g Sugar 5 g Protein 7 g Cholesterol 16 mg

213.Deep-dish Giant Double Chocolate Chip Cookie

Ingredients:
- 1 large egg
- 1 cup all-purpose flour
- ½ tsp baking powder
- ½ tsp salt
- 1 cup chocolate chip
- ½ cup unsalted butter
- ½ cup light brown sugar
- ½ cup white sugar
- 1 tsp vanilla
- ½ cup chocolate chunks

Directions:
1. Preheat oven to 350°F.
2. Melt butter in oven over low heat.
3. Add sugars and stir well.
4. Incorporate vanilla and egg, and beat quickly to make sure eggs do not cook.
5. Stir in flour, baking soda and salt.
6. Fold in chocolate chips and chunks and spread dough out in oven lightly with a spatula to flatten.
7. Bake for 25 minutes until cookie appears browned on top.

214.Turkey Bacon-wrapped Dates

Servings: 16 Appetizers
Cooking Time: 6 Minutes
Ingredients:
- 16 whole dates, pitted
- 16 whole almonds
- 6 to 8 strips turkey bacon, cut in half
- Special Equipment:
- 16 toothpicks, soaked in water for at least 30 minutes

Directions:
1. On a flat work surface, stuff each pitted date with a whole almond.
2. Wrap half slice of bacon around each date and secure it with a toothpick.
3. Place the bacon-wrapped dates in the air fryer basket.
4. Put the air fryer basket on the baking pan and slide into Rack Position 2, select Air Fry, set temperature to 390ºF (199ºC), and set time to 6 minutes.
5. When cooking is complete, transfer the dates to a paper towel-lined plate to drain. Serve hot.

215.Orange And Anise Cake

Servings: 6
Cooking Time: 20 Minutes
Ingredients:
- 1 stick butter, at room temperature
- 5 tablespoons liquid monk fruit
- 2 eggs plus 1 egg yolk, beaten
- $1/3$ cup hazelnuts, roughly chopped
- 3 tablespoons sugar-free orange marmalade
- 6 ounces (170 g) unbleached almond flour
- 1 teaspoon baking soda
- ½ teaspoon baking powder
- ½ teaspoon ground cinnamon
- ½ teaspoon ground allspice
- ½ ground anise seed
- Cooking spray

Directions:
1. Lightly spritz the baking pan with cooking spray.

2. In a mixing bowl, whisk the butter and liquid monk fruit until the mixture is pale and smooth. Mix in the beaten eggs, hazelnuts, and marmalade and whisk again until well incorporated.
3. Add the almond flour, baking soda, baking powder, cinnamon, allspice, anise seed and stir to mix well.
4. Scrape the batter into the prepared baking pan.
5. Slide the baking pan into Rack Position 1, select Convection Bake, set temperature to 310ºF (154ºC), and set time to 20 minutes.
6. When cooking is complete, the top of the cake should spring back when gently pressed with your fingers.
7. Transfer to a wire rack and let the cake cool to room temperature. Serve immediately.

216.Churros With Chocolate Dipping Sauce

Servings: 4
Cooking Time: 10 Minutes
Ingredients:
- 1 ½ cup water, divided
- ¼ cup + 1 tsp butter, unsalted
- ¼ cup + 1 tsp sugar
- 1 cup flour
- 2 eggs
- 1/8 tsp salt
- 1 cup dark chocolate (60-70% cocoa solids), chopped

Directions:
1. Lightly spray baking pan with cooking spray.
2. In a saucepan, combine 1 cup water, ¼ cup butter, and 1 teaspoon sugar. Cook over medium heat until butter has melted, stirring frequently.
3. Add the flour and stir quickly to form a loose paste. Reduce heat to low and cook, stirring, until mixture starts to come away from sides of pan and firm up. Remove from heat and let cool 10 minutes.
4. Beat in eggs and salt until combined, mixture should be smooth and glossy. Transfer to a pastry bag fitted with a star shaped nozzle.
5. Pipe mixture into any shape desired on the baking pan. Place the pan in position 2 and set oven to air fry on 390°F for 6 minutes. Cook until crisp and golden brown. Repeat with remaining batter.
6. Place the chocolate, remaining water, and sugar in a double boiler. Let sit until chocolate and sugar melts completely, stirring occasionally.
7. When the mixture is melted and smooth, stir in butter and continue cooking until melted and combined. Serve immediately with churros.
Nutrition Info: Calories 638, Total Fat 36g, Saturated Fat 20g, Total Carbs 66g, Net Carbs 61g,

Protein 10g, Sugar 33g, Fiber 5g, Sodium 211mg, Potassium 393mg, Phosphorus 234mg

217.Banana Clafouti

Ingredients:
- 1 tsp vanilla extract
- 2 Tbsp butter, melted
- ¼ tsp salt
- ½ cup all-purpose flour
- 2 bananas, peeled and thinly sliced
- 2 tsp fresh lemon juice
- 1 cup whole milk
- ¼ cup whipping cream
- 3 eggs
- ½ cup granulated sugar

Directions:
1. Preheat the oven to 350°F.
2. Whisk together milk, cream, eggs, sugar, extract, butter and salt.
3. Add the flour and whisk gently until incorporated.
4. Place sliced bananas in a bowl with lemon juice.
5. Lightly grease oven and heat in oven for 5 minutes. Remove and pour in batter.
6. Scatter bananas over batter and bake until golden and puffed, about 35 minutes.

218.Vanilla Chocolate Chip Cookies

Servings: 30 Cookies
Cooking Time: 22 Minutes
Ingredients:
- $1/3$ cup (80g) organic brown sugar
- $1/3$ cup (80g) organic cane sugar
- 4 ounces (112g) cashew-based vegan butter
- ½ cup coconut cream
- 1 teaspoon vanilla extract
- 2 tablespoons ground flaxseed
- 1 teaspoon baking powder
- 1 teaspoon baking soda
- Pinch of salt
- 2¼ cups (220g) almond flour
- ½ cup (90g) dairy-free dark chocolate chips

Directions:
1. Line the baking pan with parchment paper.
2. Mix together the brown sugar, cane sugar, and butter in a medium bowl or the bowl of a stand mixer. Cream together with a mixer.
3. Fold in the coconut cream, vanilla, flaxseed, baking powder, baking soda, and salt. Stir well.
4. Add the almond flour, a little at a time, mixing after each addition until fully incorporated. Stir in the chocolate chips with a spatula.
5. Scoop the dough into the prepared baking pan.

6. Slide the baking pan into Rack Position 1, select Convection Bake, set temperature to 325°F (160°C), and set the time to 22 minutes.
7. Bake until the cookies are golden brown.
8. When cooking is complete, transfer the baking pan onto a wire rack to cool completely before serving.

219.Hot Coconut 'n Cocoa Buns

Servings: 8
Cooking Time: 15 Minutes
Ingredients:
- Eggs, 4.
- Coconut flour, 1/3 cup
- Cacao powder, 3 tbsps.
- Coconut milk, 1 cup
- Cacao nibs, ¼ cup

Directions:
1. Preheat the air fryer for 5 minutes.
2. Combine all ingredients in a mixing bowl.
3. Form buns using your hands and place in a baking dish that will fit in the air fryer.
4. Bake for 15 minutes for 375F.
5. Once air fryer turns off, leave the buns in the air fryer until it cools completely.
Nutrition Info: Calories: 161 Carbs: 4g Protein: 5.7g Fat: 13.6g

220.Caramelized Peaches

Servings: 4
Cooking Time: 10 To 13 Minutes
Ingredients:
- 2 tablespoons sugar
- ¼ teaspoon ground cinnamon
- 4 peaches, cut into wedges
- Cooking spray

Directions:
1. Toss the peaches with the sugar and cinnamon in a medium bowl until evenly coated.
2. Lightly spray the air fryer basket with cooking spray. Place the peaches in the basket in a single layer. Lightly mist the peaches with cooking spray.
3. Put the air fryer basket on the baking pan and slide into Rack Position 2, select Air Fry, set temperature to 350ºF (180ºC), and set time to 10 minutes.
4. After 5 minutes, remove from the oven and flip the peaches. Return to the oven and continue cooking for 5 minutes.
5. When cooking is complete, the peaches should be caramelized. If necessary, continue cooking for 3 minutes. Remove from the oven. Let the peaches cool for 5 minutes and serve warm.

221.Currant Pudding

Servings: 6
Cooking Time: 15 Minutes
Ingredients:
- 1 cup red currants, blended
- 1 cup coconut cream
- 1 cup black currants, blended
- 3 tbsp. stevia

Directions:
1. In a bowl, combine all the ingredients and stir well.
2. Divide into ramekins, put them in the fryer and cook at 340°F for 20 minutes
3. Serve the pudding cold.
Nutrition Info: Calories: 200; Fat: 4g; Fiber: 2g; Carbs: 4g; Protein: 6g

222.Choco Cookies

Servings: 8
Cooking Time: 8 Minutes
Ingredients:
- 3 egg whites
- 3/4 cup cocoa powder, unsweetened
- 1 3/4 cup confectioner sugar
- 1 1/2 tsp vanilla

Directions:
1. Fit the oven with the rack in position
2. In a mixing bowl, whip egg whites until fluffy soft peaks. Slowly add in cocoa, sugar, and vanilla.
3. Drop teaspoonful onto parchment-lined baking pan into 32 small cookies.
4. Set to bake at 350 F for 8 minutes. After 5 minutes place the baking pan in the preheated oven.
5. Serve and enjoy.
Nutrition Info: Calories 132 Fat 1.1 g Carbohydrates 31 g Sugar 0.3 g Protein 2 g Cholesterol 0 mg

223.Crunchy Parmesan And Garlic Zucchini

Ingredients:
- 1 cup panko crumbs, seasoned with salt, pepper and paprika
- 1 cup freshly grated parmesan
- 3 Tbsp olive oil
- 4-6 small green zucchini, sliced into spears by cutting into ½
- lengthwise and then into thirds
- Coarse salt and pepper, to taste
- 4 garlic cloves, sliced thin

Directions:
1. Preheat oven to 450°F.

2.   Heat oil in a large oven on medium-low heat.
3.   Add zucchini and let brown on one side for 3 minutes and flip over pieces. Cook for another 3 minutes.
4.   Sprinkle with salt and pepper.
5.   Add sliced garlic and saute for 1 minute.
6.   Sprinkle panko crumbs and grated cheese on top.
7.   Transfer to oven until brown and bubbly, about 5-10 minutes.

224.Crack Dip

Servings: 15
Cooking Time: 15 Minutes
Ingredients:
- 8 oz cream cheese
- 1/8 tsp cayenne
- 1/3 cup green onion, chopped
- 1/3 cup bacon bits, cooked
- 1/3 cup sour cream
- ¾ cup ranch dressing

Directions:
1.   Fit the oven with the rack in position 2.
2.   Add all ingredients into the bowl and mix well and pour into the greased baking dish.
3.   Set to bake at 350 F for 20 minutes. After 5 minutes place the baking dish in the preheated oven.
4.   Serve and enjoy.
Nutrition Info: Calories 168 Fat 16 g Carbohydrates 1 g Sugar 0 g Protein 3 g Cholesterol 8 mg

225.Easy Ricotta Cake

Servings: 8
Cooking Time: 45 Minutes
Ingredients:
- 2 eggs
- 1/2 cup erythritol
- 1/4 cup coconut flour
- 15 oz ricotta
- Pinch of salt

Directions:
1.   Fit the oven with the rack in position
2.   In a bowl whisk eggs.
3.   Add remaining ingredients and mix until well combined.
4.   Transfer batter in greased cake pan.
5.   Set to bake at 350 F for 50 minutes. After 5 minutes place the cake pan in the preheated oven.
6.   Slice and serve.
Nutrition Info: Calories 91 Fat 5.4 g Carbohydrates 3.1 g Sugar 0.3 g Protein 7.5 g Cholesterol 57 mg

226.Choco – Chip Muffins

Ingredients:
- 3 tsp. vinegar
- ½ cup chocolate chips
- ½ tsp. vanilla essence
- Muffin cups or butter paper cups
- 2 cups All-purpose flour
- 1 ½ cup milk
- ½ tsp. baking powder
- ½ tsp. baking soda
- 2 tbsp. butter
- 1 cup sugar

Directions:
1.   Mix the ingredients together and use your Oregano Fingers to get a crumbly mixture.
2.   Add the baking soda and the vinegar to the milk and mix continuously. Add this milk to the mixture and create a batter, which you will need to transfer to the muffin cups.
3.   Preheat the fryer to 300 Fahrenheit for five minutes. You will need to place the muffin cups in the basket and cover it. Cook the muffins for fifteen minutes and check whether or not the muffins are cooked using a toothpick.
4.   Remove the cups and serve hot.

227.Old Bay Chicken Wings

Servings: 4
Cooking Time: 13 Minutes
Ingredients:
- 2 tablespoons Old Bay seasoning
- 2 teaspoons baking powder
- 2 teaspoons salt
- 2 pounds (907 g) chicken wings, patted dry
- Cooking spray

Directions:
1.   Combine the Old Bay seasoning, baking powder, and salt in a large zip-top plastic bag. Add the chicken wings, seal, and shake until the wings are thoroughly coated in the seasoning mixture.
2.   Lightly spray the air fryer basket with cooking spray. Lay the chicken wings in the basket in a single layer and lightly mist them with cooking spray.
3.   Put the air fryer basket on the baking pan and slide into Rack Position 2, select Air Fry, set temperature to 400ºF (205ºC), and set time to 13 minutes.
4.   Flip the wings halfway through the cooking time.
5.   When cooking is complete, the wings should reach an internal temperature of 165ºF (74ºC) on a meat thermometer. Remove from the oven to a plate and serve hot.

228.Spicy Snack Mix

Ingredients:

- ½ cup butter, melted
- 3 tablespoons Worcestershire sauce
- 2 teaspoons dried Italian seasoning
- ½ teaspoon crushed red pepper flakes
- 2 cups salted mixed nuts
- 2 cups small pretzels
- 2 cups potato sticks
- teaspoon white pepper

Directions:

1. Preheat oven to 300ºF. Pour nuts, pretzels, and potato sticks onto two cookie sheets with sides. In small saucepan, combine melted butter with remaining ingredients. Drizzle over the nut mixture. Toss to coat. Bake at 300ºF for 20 to 25 minutes, or until mixture is glazed and fragrant, stirring once during baking.
2. Cool snack mix and pack into zipper-lock bags. Label bags and freeze.
3. To thaw and reheat: Thaw at room temperature for 1 to 3 hours. Spread on baking sheet and reheat in 300ºF oven for 5 to 8 minutes, until crisp.

MEAT RECIPES

229.Simple Jerk Chicken Wings

Servings: 2
Cooking Time: 20 Minutes
Ingredients:
- 1 lb chicken wings
- 1 tbsp jerk seasoning
- 1 tsp olive oil
- 1 tbsp cornstarch
- Pepper
- Salt

Directions:
1. Fit the oven with the rack in position 2.
2. In a large bowl, add chicken wings.
3. Add remaining ingredients on top of chicken wings and toss to coat.
4. Add chicken wings to the air fryer basket then place an air fryer basket in the baking pan.
5. Place a baking pan on the oven rack. Set to air fry at 380 F for 20 minutes.
6. Serve and enjoy.
Nutrition Info: Calories 466 Fat 19.1 g Carbohydrates 3.7 g Sugar 0 g Protein 65.6 g Cholesterol 202 mg

230.Chicken Oregano Fingers

Ingredients:
- 1 lb. boneless chicken breast cut into Oregano Fingers
- 2 cup dry breadcrumbs
- 2 tsp. oregano
- 1 ½ tbsp. ginger-garlic paste
- 4 tbsp. lemon juice
- 2 tsp. salt
- 1 tsp. pepper powder
- 1 tsp. red chili powder
- 6 tbsp. corn flour
- 4 eggs

Directions:
1. Mix all the ingredients for the marinade and put the chicken Oregano Fingers inside and let it rest overnight.
2. Mix the breadcrumbs, oregano and red chili flakes well and place the marinated Oregano Fingers on this mixture. Cover it with plastic wrap and leave it till right before you serve to cook.
3. Pre heat the oven at 160 degrees Fahrenheit for 5 minutes. Place the Oregano Fingers in the fry basket and close it. Let them cook at the same temperature for another 15 minutes or so. Toss the Oregano Fingers well so that they are cooked uniformly.

231.Garlic-buttery Chicken Wings

Servings: 4
Cooking Time: 20 Minutes
Ingredients:
- 12 chicken wings
- ¼ cup butter
- ¼ cup honey
- ½ tbsp salt
- 4 garlic cloves, minced
- ¾ cup potato starch

Directions:
1. Preheat on Air Fry function to 370 F. Coat chicken with potato starch. Transfer to the greased Air Fryer basket and fit in the baking tray. Cook for 5 minutes. Whisk the rest of the ingredients in a bowl. Pour the sauce over the wings and serve.

232.Spanish Chicken And Pepper Baguette

Servings: 2
Cooking Time: 20 Minutes
Ingredients:
- 1¼ pounds (567 g) assorted small chicken parts, breasts cut into halves
- ¼ teaspoon salt
- ¼ teaspoon ground black pepper
- 2 teaspoons olive oil
- ½ pound (227 g) mini sweet peppers
- ¼ cup light mayonnaise
- ¼ teaspoon smoked paprika
- ½ clove garlic, crushed
- Baguette, for serving
- Cooking spray

Directions:
1. Spritz the air fryer basket with cooking spray.
2. Toss the chicken with salt, ground black pepper, and olive oil in a large bowl.
3. Arrange the sweet peppers and chicken in the basket.
4. Put the air fryer basket on the baking pan and slide into Rack Position 2, select Air Fry, set temperature to 375ºF (190ºC) and set time to 20 minutes.
5. Flip the chicken and transfer the peppers on a plate halfway through.
6. When cooking is complete, the chicken should be well browned.
7. Meanwhile, combine the mayo, paprika, and garlic in a small bowl. Stir to mix well.
8. Assemble the baguette with chicken and sweet pepper, then spread with mayo mixture and serve.

233.Mom's Meatballs

Servings: 4
Cooking Time: 20 Minutes
Ingredients:
- 1 lb ground beef
- 2 tbsp olive oil
- 1 red onion, chopped
- 1 garlic clove, minced
- 2 whole eggs, beaten
- Salt and black pepper to taste

Directions:
1. Warm olive oil in a pan over medium heat and sauté onion and garlic for 3 minutes until tender; transfer to a bowl. Add in ground beef and egg and mix well. Season with salt and pepper.
2. Preheat Breville oven to 360 F on AirFry function. Mold the mixture into golf-size ball shapes. Place the balls in the greased frying basket and cook for 12-14 minutes. Serve.

234.Bacon-wrapped Sausage With Tomato Relish

Servings: 4
Cooking Time: 32 Minutes
Ingredients:
- 8 pork sausages
- 8 bacon strips
- Relish:
- 8 large tomatoes, chopped
- 1 small onion, peeled
- 1 clove garlic, peeled
- 1 tablespoon white wine vinegar
- 3 tablespoons chopped parsley
- 1 teaspoon smoked paprika
- 2 tablespoons sugar
- Salt and ground black pepper, to taste

Directions:
1. Purée the tomatoes, onion, and garlic in a food processor until well mixed and smooth.
2. Pour the purée in a saucepan and drizzle with white wine vinegar. Sprinkle with salt and ground black pepper. Simmer over medium heat for 10 minutes.
3. Add the parsley, paprika, and sugar to the saucepan and cook for 10 more minutes or until it has a thick consistency. Keep stirring during the cooking. Refrigerate for an hour to chill.
4. Wrap the sausage with bacon strips and secure with toothpicks, then place them in the basket.
5. Put the air fryer basket on the baking pan and slide into Rack Position 2, select Air Fry, set temperature to 350ºF (180ºC) and set time to 12 minutes.

6. Flip the bacon-wrapped sausage halfway through.
7. When cooking is complete, the bacon should be crispy and browned.
8. Transfer the bacon-wrapped sausage on a plate and baste with the relish or just serve with the relish alongside.

235.Baked Zucchini Chicken Tenders

Servings: 4
Cooking Time: 30 Minutes
Ingredients:
- 2 lbs chicken tenders
- 1 large zucchini
- 2 tbsp feta cheese, crumbled
- 1 tbsp fresh lemon juice
- 1 tbsp fresh dill, chopped
- 1 cup grape tomatoes
- 2 tbsp olive oil

Directions:
1. Fit the oven with the rack in position
2. Coat chicken with oil and place in baking pan along with zucchini, dill, and tomatoes. Season with salt.
3. Set to bake at 400 F for 35 minutes. After 5 minutes place the baking dish in the preheated oven.
4. Drizzle with lemon juice and top with feta cheese.
5. Serve and enjoy.
Nutrition Info: Calories 527 Fat 25.1 g Carbohydrates 5.2 g Sugar 2.9 g Protein 67.9 g Cholesterol 206 mg

236.Pork Chops With Potatoes(2)

Servings: 6
Cooking Time: 25 Minutes
Ingredients:
- 6 pork chops
- 1 oz dried Italian dressing
- 1/4 cup olive oil
- 1 onion, chopped
- 1 lb baby potatoes, quartered
- Pepper
- Salt

Directions:
1. Fit the oven with the rack in position
2. Brush pork chops with oil and season with pepper and salt.
3. Place pork chops into the baking dish.
4. Toss potatoes, onion, and Italian dressing in a bowl and place potatoes and onion around the pork chops in baking dish.

5. Set to bake at 425 F for 30 minutes. After 5 minutes place the baking dish in the preheated oven.
6. Serve and enjoy.
Nutrition Info: Calories 393 Fat 29.7 g Carbohydrates 11.6 g Sugar 1.2 g Protein 20.1 g Cholesterol 72 mg

237.Gold Cutlets With Aloha Salsa

Servings: 4
Cooking Time: 7 Minutes
Ingredients:
- 2 eggs
- 2 tablespoons milk
- ¼ cup all-purpose flour
- ¼ cup panko bread crumbs
- 4 teaspoons sesame seeds
- 1 pound (454 g) boneless, thin pork cutlets (½-inch thick)
- ¼ cup cornstarch
- Salt and ground lemon pepper, to taste
- Cooking spray
- Aloha Salsa:
- 1 cup fresh pineapple, chopped in small pieces
- ¼ cup red bell pepper, chopped
- ½ teaspoon ground cinnamon
- 1 teaspoon soy sauce
- ¼ cup red onion, finely chopped
- ⅛ teaspoon crushed red pepper
- ⅛ teaspoon ground black pepper

Directions:
1. In a medium bowl, stir together all ingredients for salsa. Cover and refrigerate while cooking the pork.
2. Beat together eggs and milk in a large bowl. In another bowl, mix the flour, panko, and sesame seeds. Pour the cornstarch in a shallow dish.
3. Sprinkle pork cutlets with lemon pepper and salt. Dip pork cutlets in cornstarch, egg mixture, and then panko coating. Spritz both sides with cooking spray.
4. Put the air fryer basket on the baking pan and slide into Rack Position 2, select Air Fry, set the temperature to 400ºF (205ºC) and set the time to 7 minutes.
5. After 3 minutes, remove from the oven. Flip the cutlets with tongs. Return to the oven and continue cooking.
6. When cooking is complete, the pork should be crispy and golden brown on both sides.
7. Serve the fried cutlets with the Aloha salsa on the side.

238.Lemony Pork Loin Chop Schnitzel

Servings: 4
Cooking Time: 15 Minutes
Ingredients:
- 4 thin boneless pork loin chops
- 2 tablespoons lemon juice
- ½ cup flour
- ¼ teaspoon marjoram
- 1 teaspoon salt
- 1 cup panko bread crumbs
- 2 eggs
- Lemon wedges, for serving
- Cooking spray

Directions:
1. On a clean work surface, drizzle the pork chops with lemon juice on both sides.
2. Combine the flour with marjoram and salt on a shallow plate. Pour the bread crumbs on a separate shallow dish. Beat the eggs in a large bowl.
3. Dredge the pork chops in the flour, then dunk in the beaten eggs to coat well. Shake the excess off and roll over the bread crumbs. Arrange the pork chops in the basket and spritz with cooking spray.
4. Put the air fryer basket on the baking pan and slide into Rack Position 2, select Air Fry, set temperature to 400ºF (205ºC) and set time to 15 minutes.
5. After 7 minutes, remove from the oven. Flip the pork. Return to the oven and continue cooking.
6. When cooking is complete, the pork should be crispy and golden.
7. Squeeze the lemon wedges over the fried chops and serve immediately.

239.Ham & Cheese Stuffed Chicken Breasts

Servings: 4
Cooking Time: 40 Minutes
Ingredients:
- 4 skinless and boneless chicken breasts
- 4 slices ham
- 4 slices Swiss cheese
- 3 tbsp all-purpose flour
- 4 tbsp butter
- 1 tbsp paprika
- 1 tbsp chicken bouillon granules
- ½ cup dry white wine
- 1 cup heavy whipping cream

Directions:
1. Preheat on Air Fry function to 380 F. Pound the chicken breasts and top with a slice of ham and Swiss cheese. Fold the edges of the chicken over the filling and secure the borders with toothpicks. In a medium bowl, combine the paprika and flour and coat in the

chicken rolls. Fry the chicken in your for 20 minutes, turning once.
2.   In a large skillet over low heat, melt the butter and add the heavy cream, bouillon granules, and wine; bring to a boil. Add in the chicken and let simmer for around 5-10 minutes. Serve.

240.Chicken With Avocado & Radish Bowl

Servings: 2
Cooking Time: 20 Minutes
Ingredients:
- 2 chicken breasts
- 1 avocado, sliced
- 4 radishes, sliced
- 1 tbsp chopped parsley
- Salt and black pepper to taste

Directions:
1.   Preheat on Air Fry function to 300 F. Cut the chicken into small cubes. Combine all ingredients in a bowl and transfer to the Air Fryer pan. Cook for 14 minutes, shaking once. Serve with cooked rice or fried red kidney beans.

241.Cheesy Chicken Escallops

Servings: 4
Cooking Time: 10 Minutes
Ingredients:
- 4 skinless chicken breasts
- 2 ½ oz panko breadcrumbs
- 1 ounce Parmesan cheese, grated
- 6 sage leaves, chopped
- 1 ¼ ounces flour
- 2 beaten eggs

Directions:
1.   Place the chicken breasts between a cling film, beat well using a rolling pin until a ½ inch thickness is achieved.
2.   In a bowl, add Parmesan cheese, sage, and breadcrumbs. Dredge the chicken into the seasoned flour and then into the eggs. Finally, coat in the breadcrumbs.
3.   Spray the chicken breasts with cooking spray and cook in your oven for 14-16 minutes at 350 F on Air Fry function.

242.Mustard Chicken Thighs

Servings: 4
Cooking Time: 50 Minutes
Ingredients:
- 1 1/2 lbs chicken thighs, skinless and boneless
- 2 tbsp Dijon mustard
- 1/4 cup French mustard

- 1/4 cup maple syrup
- 1 tbsp olive oil

Directions:
1.   Fit the oven with the rack in position
2.   In a bowl, mix maple syrup, olive oil, Dijon mustard, and French mustard.
3.   Add chicken to the bowl and coat well.
4.   Arrange chicken in a baking dish.
5.   Set to bake at 375 F for 55 minutes. After 5 minutes place the baking dish in the preheated oven.
6.   Serve and enjoy.
Nutrition Info: Calories 410 Fat 16.5 g Carbohydrates 13.6 g Sugar 11.8 g Protein 49.6 g Cholesterol 151 mg

243.Sweet Chinese Chicken Wingettes

Servings: 4
Cooking Time: 25 Minutes
Ingredients:
- 1 lb chicken wingettes
- 1 tbsp fresh cilantro, chopped
- Salt and black pepper to taste
- 1 tbsp roasted peanuts, chopped
- ½ tbsp apple cider vinegar
- 1 garlic clove, minced
- ½ tbsp chili sauce
- 1 ginger, minced
- 1 ½ tbsp soy sauce
- 2 ½ tbsp honey

Directions:
1.   Season chicken with salt and black pepper. In a bowl, mix ginger, garlic, chili sauce, honey, soy sauce, cilantro, and vinegar. Cover chicken with honey sauce. Place the prepared chicken in the basket and cook for 20 minutes at 360 F on AirFry function. Serve sprinkled with peanuts.

244.Bacon Ranch Chicken

Servings: 6
Cooking Time: 45 Minutes
Ingredients:
- 2 lbs chicken breasts
- 1 packet dry ranch dressing mix
- 2 cups cheddar cheese, shredded
- 1 tsp garlic powder
- 4 oz cream cheese
- 1 cup sour cream
- 12 oz broccoli, steam
- 1 lb bacon, cooked & chopped

Directions:
1.   Fit the oven with the rack in position
2.   Place chicken breasts and broccoli into the greased baking pan.

3. Mix together sour cream, cream cheese, garlic powder, bacon, and ranch dressing mix and pour over chicken and broccoli.
4. Sprinkle cheddar cheese on top of chicken and broccoli mixture.
5. Set to bake at 350 F for 50 minutes. After 5 minutes place the baking pan in the preheated oven.
6. Serve and enjoy.
Nutrition Info: Calories 844 Fat 60.8 g Carbohydrates 11.8 g Sugar 1.5 g Protein 65.6 g Cholesterol 212 mg

245.Popcorn Turkey

Servings: 4
Cooking Time: 10 Minutes
Ingredients:
- Nonstick cooking spray
- 1 cup flour
- 2 eggs
- ½ cup milk
- 2 tbsp. Cajun seasoning
- 2 cups bread crumbs
- 1 large turkey breast, cut in 1-inch pieces

Directions:
1. Place the baking pan in position 2 of the oven. Lightly spray the fryer basket with cooking spray.
2. In a large bowl, whisk together flour, eggs, milk, and seasoning.
3. Place bread crumbs in a shallow dish.
4. Add the turkey to the batter and stir to coat. Roll each piece of turkey in the bread crumbs and place them in the fryer basket, these may need to be cooked in batches. Spray them lightly with cooking spray.
5. Place the basket in the oven and set to air fry on 375°F for 10 minutes. Cook turkey nuggets until crisp and golden brown, turning over halfway through cooking time. Serve with your favorite dipping sauce.
Nutrition Info: Calories 655, Total Fat 11g, Saturated Fat 3g, Total Carbs 64g, Net Carbs 61g, Protein 78g, Sugar 5g, Fiber 3g, Sodium 690mg, Potassium 855mg, Phosphorus 744mg

246.Guacamole Stuffed Chicken

Servings: 4
Cooking Time: 10 Minutes
Ingredients:
- Nonstick cooking spray
- 2 chicken breasts, boneless & skinless
- ½ cup guacamole
- 2/3 cup cheddar cheese, grated
- 1 cup panko bread crumbs
- ½ tsp Adobo seasoning

Directions:
1. Place baking pan in position 2. Spray the fryer basket with cooking spray.
2. Cut the chicken breasts in half, similar to butterflying them but cut all the way through. Place the chicken between two sheets of plastic wrap and pound really thin.
3. Spread 2 tablespoons guacamole over each piece of chicken. Sprinkle with the cheese. Fold the chicken pieces in half covering the filling.
4. In a shallow dish, combine bread crumbs and seasoning. Coat each side of chicken with mixture and place in the fryer basket.
5. Place the basket in the oven and set to air fry on 375°F for 10 minutes. Turn chicken over halfway through cooking time. Serve immediately.
Nutrition Info: Calories 363, Total Fat 15g, Saturated Fat 5g, Total Carbs 22g, Net Carbs 19g, Protein 35g, Sugar 2g, Fiber 3g, Sodium 441mg, Potassium 604mg, Phosphorus 400mg

247.Apricot-glazed Chicken Drumsticks

Servings: 6 Drumsticks
Cooking Time: 30 Minutes
Ingredients:
- For the Glaze:
- ½ cup apricot preserves
- ½ teaspoon tamari
- ¼ teaspoon chili powder
- 2 teaspoons Dijon mustard
- For the Chicken:
- 6 chicken drumsticks
- ½ teaspoon seasoning salt
- 1 teaspoon salt
- ½ teaspoon ground black pepper
- Cooking spray
- Make the glaze:

Directions:
1. Combine the ingredients for the glaze in a saucepan, then heat over low heat for 10 minutes or until thickened.
2. Turn off the heat and sit until ready to use.
3. Make the Chicken:
4. Spritz the air fryer basket with cooking spray.
5. Combine the seasoning salt, salt, and pepper in a small bowl. Stir to mix well.
6. Place the chicken drumsticks in the basket. Spritz with cooking spray and sprinkle with the salt mixture on both sides.
7. Put the air fryer basket on the baking pan and slide into Rack Position 2, select Air Fry, set temperature to 370ºF (188ºC) and set time to 20 minutes.
8. Flip the chicken halfway through.

9. When cooking is complete, the chicken should be well browned.
10. Baste the chicken with the glaze and air fry for 2 more minutes or until the chicken tenderloin is glossy.
11. Serve immediately.

248.Simple Air Fried Chicken Wings

Servings: 4
Cooking Time: 15 Minutes
Ingredients:
- 1 tablespoon olive oil
- 8 whole chicken wings
- Chicken seasoning or rub, to taste
- 1 teaspoon garlic powder
- Freshly ground black pepper, to taste

Directions:
1. Grease the basket with olive oil.
2. On a clean work surface, rub the chicken wings with chicken seasoning and rub, garlic powder, and ground black pepper.
3. Arrange the well-coated chicken wings in the basket.
4. Put the air fryer basket on the baking pan and slide into Rack Position 2, select Air Fry, set temperature to 400ºF (205ºC) and set time to 15 minutes.
5. Flip the chicken wings halfway through.
6. When cooking is complete, the internal temperature of the chicken wings should reach at least 165ºF (74ºC).
7. Remove the chicken wings from the oven. Serve immediately.

249.Beef Kinking Coriander Powder

Ingredients:
- 3 tbsp. cream
- 2 tbsp. coriander powder
- 4 tbsp. fresh mint (chopped)
- 3 tbsp. chopped capsicum
- 2 tbsp. peanut flour
- 1 lb. boneless beef liver (Chop into cubes)
- 3 onions chopped
- 5 green chilies-roughly chopped
- 1 ½ tbsp. ginger paste
- 1 ½ tsp. garlic paste
- 1 ½ tsp. salt
- 3 tsp. lemon juice
- 2 tsp. garam masala
- 4 tbsp. chopped coriander
- 3 eggs

Directions:

1. Mix the dry ingredients in a bowl. Make the mixture into a smooth paste and coat the beef cubes with the mixture.
2. Beat the eggs in a bowl and add a little salt to them. Dip the cubes in the egg mixture and coat them with sesame seeds and leave them in the refrigerator for an hour. Pre heat the oven at 290 Fahrenheit for around 5 minutes.
3. Place the kebabs in the basket and let them cook for another 25 minutes at the same temperature. Turn the kebabs over in between the cooking process to get a uniform cook. Serve the kebabs with mint sauce.

250.Meatloaf(2)

Servings: 6
Cooking Time: 55 Minutes
Ingredients:
- 2 lbs ground beef
- 1/2 cup sunflower seed flour
- 1/2 cup salsa, low-fodmap
- 2 eggs, lightly beaten
- 1 tsp oregano
- 1 tsp paprika
- 1 tsp cumin
- 1/4 cup fresh cilantro, chopped
- 1/4 cup green onion, chopped
- 1 bell pepper, diced & sautéed
- 1/2 tsp salt

Directions:
1. Fit the oven with the rack in position
2. Add all ingredients into the mixing bowl and mix until well combined.
3. Pour mixture into the greased loaf pan.
4. Set to bake at 375 F for 60 minutes. After 5 minutes place the loaf pan in the preheated oven.
5. Slice and serve.
Nutrition Info: Calories 306 Fat 10.4 g Carbohydrates 3.1 g Sugar 0.9 g Protein 47.3 g Cholesterol 162 mg

251.Honey Garlic Chicken Wings

Servings: 6
Cooking Time: 50 Minutes
Ingredients:
- 3 lbs chicken wings
- 1 tbsp garlic, minced
- 1 cup honey
- 2 tbsp BBQ sauce
- 1/2 cup soy sauce
- 2 tbsp olive oil
- Pepper
- Salt

Directions:
1. Fit the oven with the rack in position
2. Add chicken wings and remaining ingredients into the mixing bowl and mix until well coated.
3. Arrange chicken wings onto the baking pan.
4. Set to bake at 350 F for 55 minutes. After 5 minutes place the baking pan in the preheated oven.
5. Serve and enjoy.

Nutrition Info: Calories 664 Fat 21.5 g Carbohydrates 50.5 g Sugar 48.1 g Protein 67.2 g Cholesterol 202 mg

252.Delicious Turkey Cutlets

Servings: 4
Cooking Time: 25 Minutes
Ingredients:
- 1 egg
- 1 1/2 lbs turkey cutlets
- 1/2 tsp garlic powder
- 1/2 tsp onion powder
- 1/2 tsp dried parsley
- 1/4 cup parmesan cheese, grated
- 1/2 cup almond flour
- 1/4 tsp pepper
- 1/2 tsp salt

Directions:
1. Fit the oven with the rack in position
2. Add egg in a small bowl and whisk well.
3. In a shallow dish, mix almond flour, parmesan cheese, parsley, onion powder, garlic powder, pepper, and salt.
4. Dip turkey cutlet into the egg and coat with almond flour mixture.
5. Place coated turkey cutlets into the baking pan.
6. Set to bake at 350 F for 30 minutes. After 5 minutes place the baking pan in the preheated oven.
7. Serve and enjoy.

Nutrition Info: Calories 346 Fat 12.6 g Carbohydrates 1.6 g Sugar 0.4 g Protein 53.9 g Cholesterol 174 mg

253.Tangy Chicken Drumsticks With Cauliflower

Servings: 4
Cooking Time: 30 Minutes
Ingredients:
- 1 lb chicken drumsticks
- ½ tsp oregano
- ¼ cup oats
- ¼ cup milk
- 1 cup cauliflower florets, steamed
- 1 egg
- 1 tbsp cayenne pepper powder

- Salt and black pepper to taste

Directions:
1. Preheat Breville on AirFry function to 350 F. Season the drumsticks with salt and pepper and rub them with the milk. Place all the other ingredients, except for the egg in a food processor.
2. Process until smooth. Dip each drumstick in the egg first, and then in the oat mixture. Arrange them on a greased baking tray. Press Start and cook in the oven for 20 minutes. Serve warm.

254.Meatloaf(3)

Servings: 8
Cooking Time: 60 Minutes
Ingredients:
- 3 eggs
- 45 Ritz crackers, crushed
- 1 1/2 lbs lean ground beef
- 1/2 cup milk
- 4 oz sharp cheddar cheese, shredded
- 1/4 cup green pepper, diced
- 1/2 cup onion, chopped
- 1/4 tsp black pepper
- 1 tsp salt
- For topping:
- 1 tsp yellow mustard
- 1/2 cup brown sugar
- 1/2 cup ketchup

Directions:
1. Fit the oven with the rack in position
2. In a small bowl, mix together all topping ingredients and set aside.
3. In a mixing bowl, beat the eggs then add cheese, green pepper, onion, cracker crumbs, milk pepper, and salt. Stir well to combine.
4. Add ground meat and mix well.
5. Make a loaf of meat mixture and place it into the parchment-lined baking pan.
6. Set to bake at 350 F for 35 minutes. After 5 minutes place the baking pan in the preheated oven.
7. Spread topping mixture on top of the meatloaf and bake for 30 minutes more.
8. Slice and serve.

Nutrition Info: Calories 316 Fat 12.7 g Carbohydrates 17 g Sugar 13.7 g Protein 32.7 g Cholesterol 154 mg

255.Steak Seared In Browned Butter

Ingredients:
- 2 (1-lb) steaks, 1 inch thick
- 1 Tbsp extra-virgin olive oil
- 3 Tbsp unsalted butter, divided

- 1 lb. Yukon gold potatoes, sliced about ½-inch thick
- 2 fresh rosemary sprigs
- Salt and freshly ground black pepper, to taste
- ½ cup beef broth

Directions:
1. Let the steaks rest at room temperature for 30 minutes.
2. In oven over medium-high heat, heat the oil and 1 Tbsp of butter.
3. Add the potatoes and rosemary and cook for 5 minutes, until fork tender. Season with salt and pepper. Remove from the pot and set aside.
4. Season the steak with salt and pepper. Add the steak to oven over high heat and cook for 5 minutes on each side for medium-rare, or longer if desired. Remove the steaks and let them rest on a cutting board.
5. Melt the remaining 2 Tbsp of butter over medium heat, stirring often. Add the broth when the butter starts to brown. Keep stirring and scraping up the browned bits using a wooden spoon.
6. Add the potatoes to the pan and heat through, about 5 minutes. Cut the steaks in half, spoon the potatoes and browned butter over each steak, and serve.

256.Dijon Roasted Lamb Chops

Servings: 4
Cooking Time: 15 Minutes
Ingredients:
- 8 lamb loin chops
- 2 tbsp. Dijon mustard
- 2 tbsp. extra virgin olive oil
- 2 cloves garlic, chopped fine
- 2 tsp dried Herbs de Provence
- ¼ tsp salt
- ¼ tsp pepper

Directions:
1. Line baking pan with parchment paper.
2. Lay chops, in a single layer, on prepared pan. Sprinkle with salt and pepper.
3. In a small bowl, combine remaining ingredients, mix well. Spoon mixture over tops of chops evenly.
4. Set oven to convection bake on 400°F for 20 minutes. After 5 minutes, place pan in position 1 of the oven and cook 15 minutes.
5. Remove from oven and let rest 5 minutes before serving.

Nutrition Info: Calories 189, Total Fat 13g, Saturated Fat 3g, Total Carbs 1g, Net Carbs 1g, Protein 17g, Sugar 0g, Fiber 0g, Sodium 296mg, Potassium 295mg, Phosphorus 170mg

257.Juicy Spicy Lemon Kebab

Ingredients:
- 2 tsp. garam masala
- 4 tbsp. chopped coriander
- 3 tbsp. cream
- 2 tbsp. coriander powder
- 4 tbsp. fresh mint (chopped)
- 3 tbsp. chopped capsicum
- 2 lb. chicken breasts cubed
- 3 onions chopped
- 5 green chilies-roughly chopped
- 1 ½ tbsp. ginger paste
- 1 ½ tsp. garlic paste
- 1 ½ tsp. salt
- 3 tsp. lemon juice
- 2 tbsp. peanut flour
- 3 eggs

Directions:
1. Mix the dry ingredients in a bowl. Make the mixture into a smooth paste and coat the chicken cubes with the mixture. Beat the eggs in a bowl and add a little salt to them. Dip the cubes in the egg mixture and coat them with sesame seeds and leave them in the refrigerator for an hour. Pre heat the oven at 290 Fahrenheit for around 5 minutes.
2. Place the kebabs in the basket and let them cook for another 25 minutes at the same temperature. Turn the kebabs over in between the cooking process to get a uniform cook. Serve the kebabs with mint sauce.

258.Parmesan Chicken Fingers With Plum Sauce

Servings: 2
Cooking Time: 20 Minutes
Ingredients:
- 2 chicken breasts, cut in strips
- 3 tbsp Parmesan cheese, grated
- ¼ tbsp fresh chives, chopped
- ⅓ cup breadcrumbs
- 1 egg white
- 2 tbsp plum sauce, optional
- ½ tbsp fresh thyme, chopped
- ½ tbsp black pepper
- 1 tbsp water

Directions:
1. Preheat on Air Fry function to 360 F. Mix the chives, Parmesan cheese, thyme, pepper and breadcrumbs. In another bowl, whisk the egg white and mix with the water. Dip the chicken strips into the egg mixture and then in the breadcrumb mixture. Place the strips in the greased basket and fit in the baking tray. Cook for 10 minutes, flipping once. Serve with plum sauce.

259.Asian Pork Shoulder

Servings: 4
Cooking Time: 15 Minutes
Ingredients:
* 1 lb pork shoulder, boneless
* 1 tbsp wine
* 1 tbsp sugar
* 2 tbsp soy sauce
* 4 tbsp honey
* 1 tsp Chinese five-spice
* 2 tsp ginger, minced
* 2 tsp garlic, minced

Directions:
1. Fit the oven with the rack in position 2.
2. Add all ingredients except pork into the large zip-lock bag and mix well.
3. Add pork and seal the bag and place it in the fridge overnight.
4. Remove pork from marinade and place in an air fryer basket then place an air fryer basket in baking pan.
5. Place a baking pan on the oven rack. Set to air fry at 390 F for 15 minutes.
6. Serve and enjoy.
Nutrition Info: Calories 419 Fat 24.3 g Carbohydrates 22.1 g Sugar 20.5 g Protein 27.1 g Cholesterol 102 mg

260.Chicken Wings With Honey & Cashew Cream

Servings: 4
Cooking Time: 25 Minutes
Ingredients:
* 2 lb chicken wings
* 1 tbsp fresh cilantro, chopped
* Salt and black pepper to taste
* 1 tbsp cashews cream
* 1 garlic clove, minced
* 1 tbsp plain yogurt
* 2 tbsp honey
* ½ tbsp white wine vinegar
* ½ tbsp ginger, minced
* ½ tbsp garlic chili sauce

Directions:
1. Preheat Breville on AirFry function to 360 F. Season the wings with salt and black pepper, place them in a baking dish. Press Start and cook for 15 minutes. In a bowl, mix the remaining ingredients. Top the chicken with sauce and cook for 5 more minutes. Serve warm.

261.Easy Baked Chicken Drumsticks

Servings: 6
Cooking Time: 45 Minutes
Ingredients:
* 6 chicken legs
* 1/4 cup Worcestershire sauce
* 2 tbsp olive oil
* 1/2 tsp paprika
* 1/2 tsp oregano
* 1 1/2 tsp onion powder
* 1 1/2 tsp garlic powder
* 1/2 tsp pepper
* 1/2 tsp salt

Directions:
1. Fit the oven with the rack in position
2. Add chicken legs and remaining ingredients into the zip-lock bag, seal bag shake well and place in the fridge for 2 hours.
3. Place marinated chicken legs in a baking pan.
4. Set to bake at 375 F for 50 minutes. After 5 minutes place the baking pan in the preheated oven.
5. Serve and enjoy.
Nutrition Info: Calories 182 Fat 9.7 g Carbohydrates 3.3 g Sugar 2.4 g Protein 19.5 g Cholesterol 59 mg

262.Easy Lamb Chops With Asparagus

Servings: 4
Cooking Time: 15 Minutes
Ingredients:
* 4 asparagus spears, trimmed
* 2 tablespoons olive oil, divided
* 1 pound (454 g) lamb chops
* 1 garlic clove, minced
* 2 teaspoons chopped fresh thyme, for serving
* Salt and ground black pepper, to taste

Directions:
1. Spritz the air fryer basket with cooking spray.
2. On a large plate, brush the asparagus with 1 tablespoon olive oil, then sprinkle with salt. Set aside.
3. On a separate plate, brush the lamb chops with remaining olive oil and sprinkle with salt and ground black pepper.
4. Arrange the lamb chops in the pan.
5. Put the air fryer basket on the baking pan and slide into Rack Position 2, select Air Fry, set temperature to 400ºF (205ºC) and set time to 15 minutes.
6. Flip the lamb chops and add the asparagus and garlic halfway through.
7. When cooking is complete, the lamb should be well browned and the asparagus should be tender.
8. Serve them on a plate with thyme on top.

263.Swedish Meatballs

Servings: 4
Cooking Time: 14 Minutes
Ingredients:
- For the meatballs
- 1 pound 93% lean ground beef
- 1 (1-ounce) packet Lipton Onion Recipe Soup & Dip Mix
- ⅓ cup bread crumbs
- 1 egg, beaten
- Salt
- Pepper
- For the gravy
- 1 cup beef broth
- ⅓ cup heavy cream
- 1 tablespoons all-purpose flour

Directions:
1. Preparing the Ingredients. In a large bowl, combine the ground beef, onion soup mix, bread crumbs, egg, and salt and pepper to taste. Mix thoroughly.
2. Using 2 tablespoons of the meat mixture, create each meatball by rolling the beef mixture around in your hands. This should yield about 10 meatballs.
3. Air Frying. Place the meatballs in the air fryer oven. It is okay to stack them. Cook for 14 minutes.
4. While the meatballs cook, prepare the gravy. Heat a saucepan over medium-high heat.
5. Add the beef broth and heavy cream. Stir for 1 to 2 minutes.
6. Add the flour and stir. Cover and allow the sauce to simmer for 3 to 4 minutes, or until thick.
7. Drizzle the gravy over the meatballs and serve.
Nutrition Info: CALORIES: 178; FAT: 14G; PROTEIN:9G; FIBER:0

264.Maple-mustard Marinaded Pork Chops

Servings: 3
Cooking Time: 30 Minutes
Ingredients:
- 3 pork chops, ½-inch thick
- Salt and black pepper to taste
- 1 tbsp maple syrup
- 1 garlic clove, minced
- 3 tbsp mustard

Directions:
1. In a bowl, add maple syrup, garlic, mustard, salt, and pepper and mix well. Add in the pork and toss to coat. Put the chops in a baking tray and place in the oven.
2. Select Bake function, adjust the temperature to 360 F, and press Start. Cook for 8-10 minutes, flip the chops, and cook further for 6 minutes. Serve with a side of steamed asparagus.

265.Bacon Broccoli Chicken

Servings: 4
Cooking Time: 30 Minutes
Ingredients:
- 4 chicken breasts, sliced in half
- 1/3 cup mozzarella cheese, shredded
- 1 cup cheddar cheese, shredded
- 1/2 cup ranch dressing
- 6 bacon slices, cooked & chopped
- 2 cups broccoli florets, chopped

Directions:
1. Fit the oven with the rack in position
2. Place chicken into the greased casserole dish.
3. Add ranch dressing, bacon, and broccoli on top of chicken.
4. Sprinkle cheddar cheese and mozzarella cheese on top of chicken.
5. Set to bake at 375 F for 35 minutes. After 5 minutes place the casserole dish in the preheated oven.
6. Serve and enjoy.
Nutrition Info: Calories 577 Fat 32.8 g Carbohydrates 5.5 g Sugar 1.7 g Protein 62.2 g Cholesterol 192 mg

266.Teriyaki Rump Steak With Broccoli And Capsicum

Servings: 4
Cooking Time: 13 Minutes
Ingredients:
- ½ pound (227 g) rump steak
- ¹/₃ cup teriyaki marinade
- 1½ teaspoons sesame oil
- ½ head broccoli, cut into florets
- 2 red capsicums, sliced
- Fine sea salt and ground black pepper, to taste
- Cooking spray

Directions:
1. Toss the rump steak in a large bowl with teriyaki marinade. Wrap the bowl in plastic and refrigerate to marinate for at least an hour.
2. Spritz the air fryer basket with cooking spray.
3. Discard the marinade and transfer the steak in the pan. Spritz with cooking spray.
4. Put the air fryer basket on the baking pan and slide into Rack Position 2, select Air Fry, set temperature to 400ºF (205ºC) and set time to 13 minutes.
5. Flip the steak halfway through.

6. When cooking is complete, the steak should be well browned.

7. Meanwhile, heat the sesame oil in a nonstick skillet over medium heat. Add the broccoli and capsicum. Sprinkle with salt and ground black pepper. Sauté for 5 minutes or until the broccoli is tender.

8. Transfer the air fried rump steak on a plate and top with the sautéed broccoli and capsicum. Serve hot.

267.Char Siu

Servings: 4
Cooking Time: 15 Minutes
Ingredients:
- ¼ cup honey
- 1 teaspoon Chinese five-spice powder
- 1 tablespoon Shaoxing wine (rice cooking wine)
- 1 tablespoon hoisin sauce
- 2 teaspoons minced garlic
- 2 teaspoons minced fresh ginger
- 2 tablespoons soy sauce
- 1 tablespoon sugar
- 1 pound (454 g) fatty pork shoulder, cut into long, 1-inch-thick pieces
- Cooking spray

Directions:
1. Combine all the ingredients, except for the pork should, in a microwave-safe bowl. Stir to mix well. Microwave until the honey has dissolved. Stir periodically.
2. Pierce the pork pieces generously with a fork, then put the pork in a large bowl. Pour in half of the honey mixture. Set the remaining sauce aside until ready to serve.
3. Press the pork pieces into the mixture to coat and wrap the bowl in plastic and refrigerate to marinate for at least 8 hours.
4. Spritz the air fryer basket with cooking spray.
5. Discard the marinade and transfer the pork pieces in the basket.
6. Put the air fryer basket on the baking pan and slide into Rack Position 2, select Air Fry, set temperature to 400ºF (205ºC) and set time to 15 minutes.
7. Flip the pork halfway through.
8. When cooking is complete, the pork should be well browned.
9. Meanwhile, microwave the remaining marinade on high for a minute or until it has a thick consistency. Stir periodically.
10. Remove the pork from the oven and allow to cool for 10 minutes before serving with the thickened marinade.

268.Meatballs(14)

Servings: 4
Cooking Time: 25 Minutes
Ingredients:
- 1 lb ground beef
- 1 tsp fresh rosemary, chopped
- 1 tbsp garlic, chopped
- 1/2 tsp pepper
- 1 tsp garlic powder
- 1 tsp onion powder
- 1/4 cup breadcrumbs
- 2 eggs
- 1 lb ground pork
- 1/2 tsp pepper
- 1 tsp sea salt

Directions:
1. Fit the oven with the rack in position
2. Add all ingredients into the mixing bowl and mix until well combined.
3. Make small balls from the meat mixture and place it into the parchment-lined baking pan.
4. Set to bake at 400 F for 30 minutes. After 5 minutes place the baking pan in the preheated oven.
5. Serve and enjoy.
Nutrition Info: Calories 441 Fat 13.7 g Carbohydrates 7.2 g Sugar 1 g Protein 68.1 g Cholesterol 266 mg

269.Honey & Garlic Chicken Drumsticks

Servings: 4
Cooking Time: 20 Minutes
Ingredients:
- 1 lb chicken drumsticks, skin removed
- 2 tbsp olive oil
- 2 tbsp honey
- 2 garlic cloves, minced

Directions:
1. Add garlic, olive oil, and honey to a sealable zip bag. Add in chicken and toss to coat. Marinate in the fridge for 30 minutes. Add the coated chicken to the frying basket and press Start. Cook for 15 minutes at 400 F on AirFry function. Serve and enjoy!

270.Shrimp Paste Chicken

Servings: 2
Cooking Time: 30 Minutes
Ingredients:
- 6 chicken wings
- ½ tbsp sugar
- 2 tbsp cornflour
- 1 tbsp white wine
- 1 tbsp shrimp paste
- 1 tbsp grated ginger

- ½ tbsp olive oil

Directions:

1. In a bowl, mix shrimp paste, olive oil, ginger, white wine, and sugar. Cover the chicken wings with the prepared marinade and roll in the flour.

2. Place the chicken in the greased baking dish and cook in your for 20 minutes at 350 F on Air Fry function. Serve.

271.Pork Fritters

Ingredients:

- 2 tbsp. garam masala
- 1 lb. sliced pork
- 3 tsp ginger finely chopped
- 1-2 tbsp. fresh coriander leaves
- 2 or 3 green chilies finely chopped
- 1 ½ tbsp. lemon juice
- Salt and pepper to taste

Directions:

1. Mix the ingredients in a clean bowl. Wet the French Cuisine Galettes slightly with water. Pre heat the oven at 160 degrees Fahrenheit for 5 minutes.

2. Place the French Cuisine Galettes in the fry basket and let them cook for another 25 minutes at the same temperature. Keep rolling them over to get a uniform cook. Serve either with mint sauce or ketchup.

272.Veal Patti With Boiled Peas

Ingredients:

- ½ lb. minced veal
- ½ cup breadcrumbs
- A pinch of salt to taste
- ½ cup of boiled peas
- ¼ tsp. ginger finely chopped
- 1 green chili finely chopped
- 1 tsp. lemon juice
- 1 tbsp. fresh coriander leaves. Chop them finely
- ¼ tsp. red chili powder
- ¼ tsp. cumin powder
- ¼ tsp. dried mango powder

Directions:

1. Take a container and into it pour all the masalas, onions, green chilies, peas, coriander leaves, lemon juice, and ginger and 1-2 tbsp. breadcrumbs. Add the minced veal as well. Mix all the ingredients well. Mold the mixture into round patties. Press them gently. Now roll them out carefully.

2. Pre heat the oven at 250 Fahrenheit for 5 minutes. Open the basket of the Fryer and arrange the patties in the basket. Close it carefully. Keep the fryer at 150 degrees for around 10 or 12 minutes. In

between the cooking process, turn the patties over to get a uniform cook. Serve hot with mint sauce.

273.Lime Chicken With Cilantro

Servings: 4
Cooking Time: 10 Minutes
Ingredients:

- 4 (4-ounce / 113-g) boneless, skinless chicken breasts
- ½ cup chopped fresh cilantro
- Juice of 1 lime
- Chicken seasoning or rub, to taste
- Salt and ground black pepper, to taste
- Cooking spray

Directions:

1. Put the chicken breasts in the large bowl, then add the cilantro, lime juice, chicken seasoning, salt, and black pepper. Toss to coat well.

2. Wrap the bowl in plastic and refrigerate to marinate for at least 30 minutes.

3. Spritz the air fryer basket with cooking spray.

4. Remove the marinated chicken breasts from the bowl and place in the basket. Spritz with cooking spray.

5. Put the air fryer basket on the baking pan and slide into Rack Position 2, select Air Fry, set temperature to 400ºF (205ºC) and set time to 10 minutes.

6. Flip the breasts halfway through.

7. When cooking is complete, the internal temperature of the chicken should reach at least 165ºF (74ºC).

8. Serve immediately.

274.Copycat Chicken Sandwich

Servings: 4
Cooking Time: 15 Minutes
Ingredients:

- 2 chicken breasts, boneless & skinless
- 1 cup buttermilk
- 1 tbsp. + 2 tsp paprika, divided
- 1 tbsp. + 1 ½ tsp garlic powder, divided
- 2 tsp salt, divided
- 2 tsp pepper, divided
- 4 brioche buns
- 1 cup flour
- ½ cup corn starch
- 1 tbsp. onion powder
- 1 tbsp. cayenne pepper
- ½ cup mayonnaise
- 1 tsp hot sauce
- Sliced pickles

Directions:

1. Place chicken between two sheets of plastic wrap and pound to ½-inch thick. Cut crosswise to get 4 cutlets.
2. In a large bowl, whisk together buttermilk and one teaspoon each paprika, garlic powder, salt, and pepper. Add chicken, cover, and refrigerate overnight.
3. Place the buns on the baking pan and place in position 2 of the oven. Set to toast for about 2-5 minutes depending how toasted you want them. Set aside.
4. In a medium shallow dish, combine flour, cornstarch, onion powder, cayenne pepper, and remaining paprika, garlic powder, salt, and pepper.
5. Whisk in 2-3 tablespoons of the buttermilk batter chicken was marinating in until smooth.
6. Lightly spray fryer basket with cooking spray.
7. Dredge chicken in the flour mixture forming a thick coating of the batter. Place in fryer basket.
8. Place basket in the oven. Set oven to air fryer on 375°F for 10 minutes. Cook until crispy and golden brown, turning chicken over halfway through cooking time.
9. In a small bowl, whisk together mayonnaise, hot sauce, 1 teaspoon paprika, and ½ teaspoon garlic powder.
10. To serve, spread top of buns with mayonnaise mixture. Place chicken on bottom buns and top with pickles then top bun.
Nutrition Info: Calories 689, Total Fat 27g, Saturated Fat 5g, Total Carbs 71g, Net Carbs 67g, Protein 38g, Sugar 7g, Fiber 4g, Sodium 1734mg, Potassium 779mg, Phosphorus 435mg

275.Herby Chicken With Lime

Servings: 4
Cooking Time: 30 Minutes + Chilling Time
Ingredients:
- 1 (2 ½ lb) whole chicken
- Salt and black pepper to taste
- 1 tbsp chili powder
- 1 tbsp garlic powder
- 4 tbsp oregano
- 2 tbsp cilantro powder
- 2 tbsp cumin powder
- 2 tbsp olive oil
- 4 tbsp paprika
- 1 lime, juiced
Directions:
1. In a bowl, pour oregano, garlic powder, chili powder, ground cilantro, paprika, cumin, pepper, salt, and olive oil. Mix well and rub the mixture onto the chicken. Refrigerate for 20 minutes.
2. Preheat on Air Fry function to 350 F. Remove the chicken from the refrigerator; place in the greased basket and fit in the baking tray; cook for 20

minutes. Use a skewer to poke the chicken to ensure that it is clear of juices. If not, cook further for 5 to 10 minutes; let it rest for 10 minutes. Drizzle lime juice all over and serve with green salad.

276.Homemade Tarragon Chicken

Servings: 4
Cooking Time: 25 Minutes
Ingredients:
- 1 lb chicken breasts
- ½ tbsp butter, melted
- Salt and black pepper to taste
- ¼ tsp dried tarragon
Directions:
1. Preheat Breville on Bake function to 380 F. Place each chicken breast on a 12x12 inches foil. Drizzle with butter and sprinkle with tarragon, salt, and pepper. Wrap the foil around the chicken in a loose way to create a flow of air. Bake for 15 minutes. Carefully unwrap and serve.

277.Easy Cajun Chicken Drumsticks

Servings: 5
Cooking Time: 18 Minutes
Ingredients:
- 1 tablespoon olive oil
- 10 chicken drumsticks
- 1½ tablespoons Cajun seasoning
- Salt and ground black pepper, to taste
Directions:
1. Grease the basket with olive oil.
2. On a clean work surface, rub the chicken drumsticks with Cajun seasoning, salt, and ground black pepper.
3. Arrange the seasoned chicken drumsticks in the basket.
4. Put the air fryer basket on the baking pan and slide into Rack Position 2, select Air Fry, set temperature to 390ºF (199ºC) and set time to 18 minutes.
5. Flip the drumsticks halfway through.
6. When cooking is complete, the drumsticks should be lightly browned.
7. Remove the chicken drumsticks from the oven. Serve immediately.

278.Sumptuous Beef And Pork Sausage Meatloaf

Servings: 4
Cooking Time: 25 Minutes
Ingredients:
- ¾ pound (340 g) ground chuck

- 4 ounces (113 g) ground pork sausage
- 2 eggs, beaten
- 1 cup Parmesan cheese, grated
- 1 cup chopped shallot
- 3 tablespoons plain milk
- 1 tablespoon oyster sauce
- 1 tablespoon fresh parsley
- 1 teaspoon garlic paste
- 1 teaspoon chopped porcini mushrooms
- ½ teaspoon cumin powder
- Seasoned salt and crushed red pepper flakes, to taste

Directions:
1. In a large bowl, combine all the ingredients until well blended.
2. Place the meat mixture in the baking pan. Use a spatula to press the mixture to fill the pan.
3. Slide the baking pan into Rack Position 1, select Convection Bake, set temperature to 360ºF (182ºC) and set time to 25 minutes.
4. When cooking is complete, the meatloaf should be well browned.
5. Let the meatloaf rest for 5 minutes. Transfer to a serving dish and slice. Serve warm.

279.Delicious Tender Chicken Breasts

Servings: 6
Cooking Time: 25 Minutes
Ingredients:
- 3 lbs chicken breasts, boneless
- 1 1/2 cups parmesan cheese, grated
- 1/2 tsp pepper
- 2 tsp garlic powder
- 1 cup sour cream
- 1 tsp salt

Directions:
1. Fit the oven with the rack in position
2. Place chicken into the baking dish.
3. In a bowl, mix 1 cup parmesan cheese, pepper, garlic powder, sour cream, and salt.
4. Pour cheese mixture over chicken and sprinkle remaining parmesan cheese on top of chicken.
5. Set to bake at 375 F for 30 minutes. After 5 minutes place the baking dish in the preheated oven.
6. Serve and enjoy.
Nutrition Info: Calories 589 Fat 29.7 g Carbohydrates 3.3 g Sugar 0.3 g Protein 74.2 g Cholesterol 235 mg

280.Spiced Pork Chops

Servings: 4
Cooking Time: 16 Minutes
Ingredients:

- 4 pork chops, boneless
- 1/2 tsp granulated onion
- 1/2 tsp granulated garlic
- 1/4 tsp sugar
- 2 tsp olive oil
- 1/2 tsp celery seed
- 1/2 tsp parsley
- 1/2 tsp salt

Directions:
1. Fit the oven with the rack in position 2.
2. Brush pork chops with olive oil.
3. Mix celery seed, parsley, granulated onion, garlic, sugar, and salt and sprinkle over pork chops.
4. Place pork chops in the air fryer basket then place an air fryer basket in the baking pan.
5. Place a baking pan on the oven rack. Set to air fry at 350 F for 16 minutes.
6. Serve and enjoy.
Nutrition Info: Calories 279 Fat 22.3 g Carbohydrates 0.6 g Sugar 0.3 g Protein 18.1 g Cholesterol 69 mg

281.Herbed Turkey Breast With Simple Dijon Sauce

Servings: 4
Cooking Time: 30 Minutes
Ingredients:
- 1 teaspoon chopped fresh sage
- 1 teaspoon chopped fresh tarragon
- 1 teaspoon chopped fresh thyme leaves
- 1 teaspoon chopped fresh rosemary leaves
- 1½ teaspoons sea salt
- 1 teaspoon ground black pepper
- 1 (2-pound / 907-g) turkey breast
- 3 tablespoons Dijon mustard
- 3 tablespoons butter, melted
- Cooking spray

Directions:
1. Spritz the air fryer basket with cooking spray.
2. Combine the herbs, salt, and black pepper in a small bowl. Stir to mix well. Set aside.
3. Combine the Dijon mustard and butter in a separate bowl. Stir to mix well.
4. Rub the turkey with the herb mixture on a clean work surface, then brush the turkey with Dijon mixture.
5. Arrange the turkey in the basket.
6. Put the air fryer basket on the baking pan and slide into Rack Position 2, select Air Fry, set temperature to 390ºF (199ºC) and set time to 30 minutes.
7. Flip the turkey breast halfway through.

8. When cooking is complete, an instant-read thermometer inserted in the thickest part of the turkey breast should reach at least 165ºF (74ºC).
9. Transfer the cooked turkey breast on a large plate and slice to serve.

282.Tender Baby Back Ribs

Servings: 4
Cooking Time: 45 Minutes
Ingredients:
- 1 rack baby back ribs, separated in 2-3 rib sections
- 1 tsp salt
- 1 tsp pepper
- 2 cloves garlic, crushed
- 1 bay leaf
- 3 tbsp. white wine
- 2 tbsp. olive oil
- 1 tsp lemon juice
- ¼ tsp paprika
- 1 tsp soy sauce
- 2 thyme stems
- Nonstick cooking spray

Directions:
1. In a large bowl, combine all ingredients, except ribs, and mix well.
2. Add ribs and turn to coat all sides. Let marinate at room temperature 30 minutes.
3. Lightly spray fryer basket with cooking spray. Place baking pan in position 1 of the oven.
4. Add ribs to basket, in a single layer, and place on baking pan. Set oven to air fry on 360°F for 45 minutes. Baste ribs with marinade and turn a few times while cooking. Serve immediately.

Nutrition Info: Calories 772, Total Fat 52g, Saturated Fat 10g, Total Carbs 2g, Net Carbs 2g, Protein 74g, Sugar 0g, Fiber 0g, Sodium 864mg, Potassium 1255mg, Phosphorus 749mg

283.Pork Sausage With Cauliflower Mash

Servings: 6
Cooking Time: 27 Minutes
Ingredients:
- 1 pound (454 g) cauliflower, chopped
- 6 pork sausages, chopped
- ½ onion, sliced
- 3 eggs, beaten
- $^1/_3$ cup Colby cheese
- 1 teaspoon cumin powder
- ½ teaspoon tarragon
- ½ teaspoon sea salt
- ½ teaspoon ground black pepper
- Cooking spray

Directions:
1. Spritz the baking pan with cooking spray.
2. In a saucepan over medium heat, boil the cauliflower until tender. Place the boiled cauliflower in a food processor and pulse until puréed. Transfer to a large bowl and combine with remaining ingredients until well blended.
3. Pour the cauliflower and sausage mixture into the pan.
4. Slide the baking pan into Rack Position 1, select Convection Bake, set temperature to 365ºF (185ºC) and set time to 27 minutes.
5. When cooking is complete, the sausage should be lightly browned.
6. Divide the mixture among six serving dishes and serve warm.

284.Pheasant Chili

Ingredients:
- 1 lb. cubed pheasant
- 2 ½ tsp. ginger-garlic paste
- 1 tsp. red chili sauce
- ¼ tsp. salt
- ¼ tsp. red chili powder/black pepper
- A few drops of edible orange food coloring
- For sauce:
- 2 tbsp. olive oil
- 1 ½ tsp. ginger garlic paste
- ½ tbsp. red chili sauce
- 2 tbsp. tomato ketchup
- 2 tsp. soya sauce
- 1-2 tbsp. honey
- ¼ tsp. Ajinomoto
- 1-2 tsp. red chili flakes

Directions:
1. Mix all the ingredients for the marinade and put the pheasant cubes inside and let it rest overnight. Mix the breadcrumbs, oregano and red chili flakes well and place the marinated Oregano Fingers on this mixture.
2. Cover it with plastic wrap and leave it till right before you serve to cook. Pre heat the oven at 160 degrees Fahrenheit for 5 minutes. Place the Oregano Fingers in the fry basket and close it. Let them cook at the same temperature for another 15 minutes or so. Toss the Oregano Fingers well so that they are cooked uniformly.

285.Delicious Coconut Chicken Casserole

Servings: 4
Cooking Time: 20 Minutes
Ingredients:
- 2 large eggs, beaten

- 2 tbsp garlic powder
- Salt and black pepper to taste
- ¾ cup breadcrumbs
- ¾ cup shredded coconut
- 1 pound chicken tenders

Directions:

1. Preheat your on Air Fry function to 400 F. Spray a baking sheet with cooking spray. In a deep dish, whisk garlic powder, eggs, pepper, and salt. In another bowl, mix the breadcrumbs and coconut. Dip your chicken tenders in egg mixture, then in the coconut mix; shake off any excess. Place the prepared chicken tenders in the greased basket and fit in the baking tray; cook for 12-14 minutes until golden brown. Serve.

APPETIZERS AND SIDE DISHES

286.Air Fried Eggplant Cubes

Servings: 2
Cooking Time: 12 Minutes
Ingredients:
- 1 eggplant, cut into cubes
- 1/4 tsp oregano
- 1 tbsp olive oil
- 1/2 tsp garlic powder

Directions:
1. Fit the oven with the rack in position 2.
2. Add all ingredients into the large bowl and toss well.
3. Transfer eggplant into in air fryer basket then places the air fryer basket in the baking pan.
4. Place a baking pan on the oven rack. Set to air fry at 390 F for 12 minutes.
5. Serve and enjoy.

Nutrition Info: Calories 120 Fat 7.4 g Carbohydrates 14.1 g Sugar 7.1 g Protein 2.4 g Cholesterol 0 mg

287.Homemade Cod Fingers

Servings: 3
Cooking Time: 25 Minutes
Ingredients:
- 2 cups flour
- Salt and black pepper to taste
- 1 tsp seafood seasoning
- 2 whole eggs, beaten
- 1 cup cornmeal
- 1 pound cod fillets, cut into fingers
- 2 tbsp milk
- 2 eggs, beaten
- 1 cup breadcrumbs
- 1 lemon, cut into wedges

Directions:
1. Preheat on Air Fryer function to 400 F. In a bowl, mix beaten eggs with milk. In a separate bowl, combine flour, cornmeal, and seafood seasoning. In another mixing bowl, mix spices with the eggs. In a third bowl, pour the breadcrumbs.
2. Dip cod fingers in the seasoned flour mixture, followed by a dip in the egg mixture, and finally coat with breadcrumbs. Place the fingers in your Air Fryer basket and fit in the baking tray. Cook for 10 minutes until golden brown. Serve with lemon wedges.

288.Poached Fennel

Servings: 3
Cooking Time: 6 Minutes
Ingredients:
- Ground nutmeg
- 1 tablespoon white flour
- 2 cups milk
- Salt, to taste
- 2 big fennel bulbs, sliced
- 2 tablespoons butter

Directions:
1. Put the Instant Pot in Saute mode, add the butter and melt. Add the fennel slices, mix and cook until lightly browned.
2. Add the flour, salt, pepper, nutmeg and milk, mix, cover and cook in the manual for 6 minutes. Relieve the pressure, transfer the fennel to the dishes and serve.

Nutrition Info: Calories: 140, Fat: 5, Fiber: 4.7, Carbohydrate: 12, Proteins: 4.4

289.Homemade French Fries

Servings: 2
Cooking Time: 25 Minutes
Ingredients:
- 2 russet potatoes, cut into strips
- 2 tbsp olive oil
- Salt and black pepper to taste

Directions:
1. In a bowl, toss the strips with olive oil and season with salt and pepper. Arrange them on the frying basket. Select AirFry function, adjust the temperature to 400 F, and press Start. Cook for 18-22 minutes. Check for crispiness and serve with aioli, ketchup, or crumbled feta cheese.

290.Mom's Tarragon Chicken Breast Packets

Servings: 2
Cooking Time: 15 Minutes
Ingredients:
- 2 chicken breasts
- 1 tbsp butter
- Salt and black pepper to taste
- ¼ tsp dried tarragon

Directions:
1. Preheat on Bake function to 380 F. Place each chicken breast on a 12x12 inches foil wrap. Top the chicken with tarragon and butter; season with salt and pepper. Wrap the foil around the chicken breast in a loose way to create a flow of air. Cook the in your oven for 15 minutes. Carefully unwrap and serve.

291.Brussels Sprouts With Garlic

Servings: 2

Cooking Time: 25 Minutes
Ingredients:
- 1 lb Brussels sprouts, trimmed
- ½ tsp garlic, chopped
- 2 tbsp olive oil
- Salt and black pepper to taste

Directions:
1. In a bowl, mix olive oil, garlic, salt, and pepper. Stir in the Brussels sprouts and let rest for 5 minutes. Place the coated sprouts in the Air Fryer basket and fit in the baking tray. Cook for 15 minutes at 380 F, shaking once. Serve warm.

292.Garlicky Roasted Chicken With Lemon

Servings: 4
Cooking Time: 60 Minutes
Ingredients:
- 1 whole chicken (around 3.5 lb)
- 1 tbsp olive oil
- Salt and black pepper to taste
- 1 lemon, cut into quarters
- 5 garlic cloves

Directions:
1. Rub the chicken with olive oil and season with salt and pepper. Stuff the cavity with lemon and garlic. Place chicken, breast-side down on a baking tray. Tuck the legs and wings tips under.
2. Select Bake function, adjust the temperature to 360 F, and press Start. Bake for 30 minutes, turn breast-side up, and bake it for another 15 minutes. Let rest for 5-6 minutes then carve.

293.Rosemary Red Potatoes

Servings: 4
Cooking Time: 20 Minutes
Ingredients:
- 1½ pounds (680 g) small red potatoes, cut into 1-inch cubes
- 2 tablespoons olive oil
- 2 tablespoons minced fresh rosemary
- 1 tablespoon minced garlic
- 1 teaspoon salt, plus additional as needed
- ½ teaspoon freshly ground black pepper, plus additional as needed

Directions:
1. Toss the potato cubes with the olive oil, rosemary, garlic, salt, and pepper in a large bowl until thoroughly coated.
2. Arrange the potato cubes in the baking pan in a single layer.
3. Slide the baking pan into Rack Position 1, select Convection Bake, set temperature to 350ºF (180ºC), and set time to 20 minutes.

4. Stir the potatoes a few times during cooking for even cooking.
5. When cooking is complete, the potatoes should be tender. Remove from the oven to a plate. Taste and add additional salt and pepper as needed.

294.Bbq Chicken Wings

Servings: 4
Cooking Time: 19 Minutes
Ingredients:
- 2 lbs. chicken wings
- 1 teaspoon olive oil
- 1 teaspoon smoked paprika
- 1 teaspoon garlic powder
- Salt and ground black pepper, as required
- ¼ cup BBQ sauce

Directions:
1. In a large bowl combine chicken wings, smoked paprika, garlic powder, oil, salt, and pepper and mix well.
2. Press "Power Button" of Air Fry Oven and turn the dial to select the "Air Fry" mode.
3. Press the Time button and again turn the dial to set the cooking time to 19 minutes.
4. Now push the Temp button and rotate the dial to set the temperature at 360 degrees F.
5. Press "Start/Pause" button to start.
6. When the unit beeps to show that it is preheated, open the lid.
7. Arrange the chicken wings in "Air Fry Basket" and insert in the oven.
8. After 12 minutes of cooking, flip the wings and coat with barbecue sauce evenly.
9. Serve immediately.
Nutrition Info: Calories 468 Total Fat 18.1 g Saturated Fat 4.8 g Cholesterol 202mg Sodium 409 mg Total Carbs 6.5 g Fiber 0.4 g Sugar 4.3 g Protein 65.8 g

295.Winter Vegetables With Herbs

Servings: 2
Cooking Time: 20 Minutes
Ingredients:
- 1/2-pound broccoli florets
- 1 celery root, peeled and cut into 1-inch pieces
- 1 onion, cut into wedges
- 2 tablespoons unsalted butter, melted
- 1/2 cup chicken broth
- 1/4 cup tomato sauce
- 1 teaspoon parsley
- 1 teaspoon rosemary
- 1 teaspoon thyme

Directions:

1. Start by preheating your Air Fryer to 380 degrees F. Place all ingredients in a lightly greased casserole dish. Stir to combine well.
2. Bake in the preheated Air Fryer for 10 minutes. Gently stir the vegetables with a large spoon and cook for 5 minutes more.
3. Serve in individual bowls with a few drizzles of lemon juice.
Nutrition Info: 141 Calories; 13g Fat; 1g Carbs; 5g Protein; 9g Sugars; 6g Fiber

296.Baked Honey Carrots

Servings: 4
Cooking Time: 25 Minutes
Ingredients:
- 1 lb baby carrots
- 2 tbsp butter, melted
- 3 tbsp honey
- 2 tsp fresh parsley, chopped
- 1 tbsp Dijon mustard
- Pepper
- Salt

Directions:
1. Fit the oven with the rack in position
2. In a large bowl, toss carrots with Dijon mustard, honey, butter, pepper, and salt.
3. Transfer carrots in a baking dish and spread evenly.
4. Set to bake at 400 F for 30 minutes. After 5 minutes place the baking dish in the preheated oven.
5. Serve and enjoy.
Nutrition Info: Calories 141 Fat 6.1 g Carbohydrates 22.6 g Sugar 18.4 g Protein 1 g Cholesterol 15 mg

297.Pumpkin Fritters With Ham & Cheese

Servings: 4
Cooking Time: 10 Minutes
Ingredients:
- ½ cup ham, chopped
- 1 cup dry pancake mix
- 1 egg
- 2 tbsp canned puree pumpkin
- 1 oz cheddar, shredded
- ½ tsp chili powder
- 3 tbsp of flour
- ½ cup beer
- 2 tbsp scallions, chopped

Directions:
1. Preheat Breville on AirFry function to 370 F. In a bowl, combine the pancake mix and chili powder. Mix in the egg, puree pumpkin, beer, cheddar cheese, ham, and scallions. Form balls and roll them in the flour.

Arrange the balls into the basket. Press Start and cook for 12 minutes.

298.Salmon Croquettes

Servings: 8
Cooking Time: 7 Minutes
Ingredients:
- ½ of large can red salmon, drained
- 1 egg, lightly beaten
- 1 tablespoon fresh parsley, chopped
- Salt and freshly ground black pepper, as needed
- 3 tablespoons vegetable oil
- ½ cup breadcrumbs

Directions:
1. In a bowl, add the salmon and with a fork, mash it completely.
2. Add the eggs, parsley, salt, and black pepper and mix until well combined.
3. Make 8 equal-sized croquettes from the mixture.
4. In a shallow dish, mix together the oil, and breadcrumbs.
5. Coat the croquettes with the breadcrumb mixture.
6. Press "Power Button" of Air Fry Oven and turn the dial to select the "Air Fry" mode.
7. Press the Time button and again turn the dial to set the cooking time to 7 minutes.
8. Now push the Temp button and rotate the dial to set the temperature at 390 degrees F.
9. Press "Start/Pause" button to start.
10. When the unit beeps to show that it is preheated, open the lid.
11. Arrange the croquettes in "Air Fry Basket" and insert in the oven.
12. Serve warm.
Nutrition Info: Calories 117 Total Fat 7.8 g Saturated Fat 1.5 g Cholesterol 33 mg Sodium 89 mg Total Carbs 4.9 g Fiber 0.3 g Sugar 0.5 g Protein 7.1 g

299.Rosemary Chickpeas

Servings: 4
Cooking Time: 20 Minutes
Ingredients:
- 2 (14.5-ounce) cans chickpeas, rinsed
- 2 tbsp olive oil
- 1 tsp dried rosemary
- ½ tsp dried thyme
- ¼ tsp dried sage
- ¼ tsp salt

Directions:
1. In a bowl, mix together chickpeas, oil, rosemary, thyme, sage, and salt. Transfer to a baking pan. Select

Bake function, adjust the temperature to 380 F, and press Start. Cook for 15 minutes.

300.Homemade Cheesy Sticks

Servings: 12
Cooking Time: 5 Minutes
Ingredients:
- 6 (6 oz) bread cheese
- 2 tbsp butter
- 2 cups panko crumbs

Directions:
1. Put the butter in a bowl and melt in the microwave for 2 minutes; set aside. With a knife, cut the cheese into equal-sized sticks. Brush each stick with butter and dip into panko crumbs. Arrange the sticks in a single layer in the basket. Fit in the baking tray and cook in the at 390 F for 10 minutes on Air Fry function. Flip halfway through. Serve warm.

301.Avocado, Tomato, And Grape Salad With Crunchy Potato Croutons

Servings: 2
Cooking Time: 10 Minutes
Ingredients:
- Potato croutons:
- 1 medium-small russet potato
- 2 cloves garlic
- 1 tablespoon extra light olive oil
- 1 tablespoon nutritional yeast
- 1/2 teaspoon garlic powder
- 1/2 teaspoon onion powder
- 1/2 teaspoon dried thyme
- 1/2 teaspoon dried rosemary
- 1/2 teaspoon dried oregano
- 1/2 teaspoon chili powder
- 1/4 teaspoon Himalayan sea salt
- 1/3 teaspoon cayenne pepper
- Pinch red pepper flakes
- Black pepper to taste
- Salad:
- 1 cup grape tomatoes
- Small handful dried cranberries
- Small handful green grapes
- 2-3 sprigs cilantro
- 1 avocado
- 2 tablespoons extra-virgin olive oil
- 1 tablespoon nutritional yeast
- 1 tablespoon lemon juice
- 1/2 teaspoon pure maple syrup
- 1/4 teaspoon salt
- Few sprinkles ground pepper
- Small handful toasted pecans

Directions:
1. Peel and cut potatoes into 1-inch cubes.
2. Place potatoes in water with a pinch of salt for 1 hour.
3. When the hour has passed, preheat the toaster oven to 450°F.
4. Drain potatoes and dry them on multiple layers of paper towels, then return to bowl.
5. Peel and mince garlic, then add to bowl.
6. Add rest of crouton ingredients to the bowl and stir together.
7. Lay potatoes mixture across a greased baking sheet in a single layer and bake for 35 minutes, flipping halfway through.
8. Combine oil, yeast, syrup, lemon juice, salt and pepper together to create salad dressing.
9. Slice tomatoes in half and put in a bowl with cranberries and grapes.
10. Chop cilantro and add to bowl. Scoop out avocado and cut it into smaller pieces and add to bowl.
11. Drizzle dressing and mix well. Add potatoes and mix again, top with pecans and serve.
Nutrition Info: Calories: 1032, Sodium: 560 mg, Dietary Fiber: 22.8 g, Total Fat: 84.9 g, Total Carbs: 64.2 g, Protein: 17.0 g.

302.Crunchy Cheese Twists

Servings: 8
Cooking Time: 45 Minutes
Ingredients:
- 2 cups cauliflower florets, steamed
- 1 egg
- 3 ½ oz oats
- 1 red onion, diced
- 1 tsp mustard
- 5 oz cheddar cheese, shredded
- Salt and black pepper to taste

Directions:
1. Preheat on Air Fry function to 350 F. Place the oats in a food processor and pulse until they are the consistency of breadcrumbs.
2. Place the cauliflower florets in a large bowl. Add in the rest of the ingredients and mix to combine. Take a little bit of the mixture and twist it into a straw.
3. Place onto a lined baking tray and repeat the process with the rest of the mixture. Cook for 10 minutes, turn over, and cook for an additional 10 minutes. Serve.

303.Crispy Cinnamon Apple Chips

Servings: 4
Cooking Time: 10 Minutes

Ingredients:
- 2 apples, cored and cut into thin slices
- 2 heaped teaspoons ground cinnamon
- Cooking spray

Directions:
1. Spritz the air fryer basket with cooking spray.
2. In a medium bowl, sprinkle the apple slices with the cinnamon. Toss until evenly coated. Spread the coated apple slices on the pan in a single layer.
3. Put the air fryer basket on the baking pan and slide into Rack Position 2, select Air Fry, set temperature to 350ºF (180ºC) and set time to 10 minutes.
4. After 5 minutes, remove from the oven. Stir the apple slices and return to the oven to continue cooking.
5. When cooking is complete, the slices should be until crispy. Remove from the oven and let rest for 5 minutes before serving.

304.Homemade Prosciutto Wrapped Cheese Sticks

Servings: 6
Cooking Time: 50 Minutes
Ingredients:
- 1 lb cheddar cheese
- 12 slices of prosciutto
- 1 cup flour
- 2 eggs, beaten
- 4 tbsp olive oil
- 1 cup breadcrumbs

Directions:
1. Cut the cheese into 6 equal sticks. Wrap each piece with 2 prosciutto slices. Place them in the freezer just enough to set. Preheat on Air Fry function to 390 F. Dip the croquettes into flour first, then in eggs, and coat with breadcrumbs. Drizzle the basket with oil and fit in the baking tray. Cook for 10 minutes or until golden. Serve.

305.Sweet Pickle Chips With Buttermilk

Servings: 3
Cooking Time: 20 Minutes
Ingredients:
- 36 sweet pickle chips
- 1 cup buttermilk
- 3 tbsp smoked paprika
- 2 cups flour
- ¼ cup cornmeal
- Salt and black pepper to taste

Directions:
1. Preheat on Air Fryer function to 400 F. In a bowl, mix flour, paprika, pepper, salt, cornmeal, and

powder. Place pickles in buttermilk and set aside for 5 minutes. Dip the pickles in the spice mixture and place them in the greased air fryer basket. Fit in the baking tray and cook for 10 minutes. Serve warm.

306.Cauliflower Mash

Servings: 4
Cooking Time: 6 Minutes
Ingredients:
- 1½ cups water
- ½ teaspoon turmeric
- 1 tablespoon butter
- 1 cauliflower, separated into florets
- Salt and ground black pepper, to taste
- 3 chives, diced

Directions:
1. Put water in the pot immediately, place the cabbage - flower in the basket for cooking, immediately cover the pot and cook 6 minutes to steam.
2. Release the pressure naturally for 2 minutes and quickly release the rest.
3. Transfer the cauliflower to a bowl and mash with a potato masher. Add salt, pepper, butter and saffron, mix, transfer to a blender and mix well. Serve with chives sprinkled on top.
Nutrition Info: Calories: 70, Fat: 5, Fiber: 2, Carbohydrate: 5, Proteins: 2

307.Rice Broccoli Casserole

Servings: 8
Cooking Time: 40 Minutes
Ingredients:
- 2 cups brown rice, cooked
- 3 cups broccoli florets
- 1 tbsp olive oil
- 2 garlic cloves, minced
- 1 onion, chopped
- For sauce:
- 1 tbsp onion, chopped
- 1/4 cup nutritional yeast flakes
- 1 cup of water
- 1 garlic clove, minced
- 1 tbsp tapioca starch
- 1 cup cashews
- 1 1/2 tsp salt

Directions:
1. Fit the oven with the rack in position
2. For the sauce: add all sauce ingredients into the blender and blend until smooth.
3. Heat oil in a pan over medium-high heat.
4. Add garlic and onion and sauté until onion is softened.

5. Add broccoli and cook for a minute.
6. Add rice and sauce and stir to combine.
7. Transfer broccoli rice mixture into the greased casserole dish.
8. Set to bake at 400 F for 45 minutes. After 5 minutes place the casserole dish in the preheated oven.
9. Serve and enjoy.
Nutrition Info: Calories 327 Fat 11.4 g Carbohydrates 49.2 g Sugar 2.1 g Protein 9.7 g Cholesterol 0 mg

308.Ham Rolls With Vegetables & Walnuts

Servings: 4
Cooking Time: 15 Minutes
Ingredients:
- 8 ham slices
- 4 carrots, chopped
- 4 slices ham
- 2 oz walnuts, finely chopped
- 1 zucchini
- 1 clove garlic
- 1 tbsp olive oil
- 1 tbsp ginger powder
- ¼ cup basil leaves, finely chopped
- Salt and black pepper to taste

Directions:
1. Heat the olive oil in a pan over medium heat and add the zucchini, carrots, garlic, ginger and salt; cook for 5 minutes. Add the basil and walnuts, and keep stirring.
2. Divide the mixture between the ham slices. Then fold one side above the filling and roll in. Cook the rolls in the preheated for 8 minutes at 300 F on Bake function.

309.Roasted Brussels Sprouts

Servings: 6
Cooking Time: 30 Minutes
Ingredients:
- 1-1/2 pounds Brussels sprouts, ends trimmed and yellow leaves removed
- 3 tablespoons olive oil
- 1 teaspoon salt
- 1/2 teaspoon black pepper

Directions:
1. Start by preheating toaster oven to 400°F.
2. Toss Brussels sprouts in a large bowl, drizzle with olive oil, sprinkle with salt and pepper, then toss.
3. Roast for 30 minutes.
Nutrition Info: Calories: 109, Sodium: 416 mg, Dietary Fiber: 4.3 g, Total Fat: 7.4 g, Total Carbs: 10.4 g, Protein: 3.9 g.

310.Japanese Tempura Bowl

Servings: 3
Cooking Time: 20 Minutes
Ingredients:
- 7 tablespoons whey protein isolate
- 1 teaspoon baking powder
- Kosher salt and ground black pepper, to taste
- 1/2 teaspoon paprika
- 1 teaspoon dashi granules
- 2 eggs
- 1 tablespoon mirin
- 3 tablespoons soda water
- 1 cup parmesan cheese, grated
- 1 onion, cut into rings
- 1 bell pepper
- 1 zucchini, cut into slices
- 3 asparagus spears
- 2 tablespoons olive oil

Directions:
1. In a shallow bowl, mix the whey protein isolate, baking powder, salt, black pepper, paprika, dashi granules, eggs, mirin, and soda water.
2. In another shallow bowl, place grated parmesan cheese.
3. Dip the vegetables in tempura batter; lastly, roll over parmesan cheese to coat evenly. Drizzle each piece with olive oil.
4. Cook in the preheated Air Fryer at 400 degrees F for 10 minutes, shaking the basket halfway through the cooking time. Work in batches until the vegetables are crispy and golden brown.
Nutrition Info: 324 Calories; 12g Fat; 5g Carbs; 26g Protein; 9g Sugars; 2g Fiber

311.Paprika Curly Potatoes

Servings: 2
Cooking Time: 20 Minutes
Ingredients:
- 2 whole potatoes, spiralized
- 1 tbsp olive oil
- Salt and black pepper to taste
- 1 tsp paprika

Directions:
1. Preheat Breville on AirFry function to 390 F.
2. Place the potatoes in a bowl and coat with oil. Transfer them to the frying basket and place in the oven. Press Start and cook for 15 minutes. Sprinkle with salt and paprika and serve.

312.Homemade Chicken Thighs

Servings: 4

Cooking Time: 30 Minutes
Ingredients:
- 1 pound chicken thighs
- ½ tsp salt
- ¼ tsp black pepper
- ¼ tsp garlic powder

Directions:
1. Season the thighs with salt, pepper, and garlic powder. Arrange them, skin side down on the frying basket. Select Bake function, adjust the temperature to 380 F, and press Start. Bake until golden brown, about 20 minutes. Serve warm.

313.Crispy Zucchini Sticks

Servings: 4
Cooking Time: 14 Minutes
Ingredients:
- 2 small zucchini, cut into 2-inch × ½-inch sticks
- 3 tablespoons chickpea flour
- 2 teaspoons arrowroot (or cornstarch)
- ½ teaspoon garlic granules
- ¼ teaspoon sea salt
- ⅛ teaspoon freshly ground black pepper
- 1 tablespoon water
- Cooking spray

Directions:
1. Combine the zucchini sticks with the chickpea flour, arrowroot, garlic granules, salt, and pepper in a medium bowl and toss to coat. Add the water and stir to mix well.
2. Spritz the air fryer basket with cooking spray and spread out the zucchini sticks in the pan. Mist the zucchini sticks with cooking spray.
3. Put the air fryer basket on the baking pan and slide into Rack Position 2, select Air Fry, set temperature to 392ºF (200ºC), and set time to 14 minutes.
4. Stir the sticks halfway through the cooking time.
5. When cooking is complete, the zucchini sticks should be crispy and nicely browned. Remove from the oven and serve warm.

314.Coriander Artichokes(2)

Servings: 4
Cooking Time: 20 Minutes
Ingredients:
- 12 oz. artichoke hearts
- 1 tbsp. lemon juice
- 1 tsp. coriander, ground
- ½ tsp. cumin seeds
- ½ tsp. olive oil
- Salt and black pepper to taste.

Directions:

1. In a pan that fits your air fryer, mix all the ingredients, toss, introduce the pan in the fryer and cook at 370°F for 15 minutes
2. Divide the mix between plates and serve as a side dish.
Nutrition Info: Calories: 200; Fat: 7g; Fiber: 2g; Carbs: 5g; Protein: 8g

315.Philly Egg Rolls

Servings: 6
Cooking Time: 25 Minutes
Ingredients:
- Nonstick cooking spray
- ½ lb. lean ground beef
- ¼ tsp garlic powder
- ¼ tsp onion powder
- ¼ tsp salt
- ¼ tsp pepper
- ¾ cup green bell pepper, chopped
- ¾ cup onion, chopped
- 2 slices provolone cheese, torn into pieces
- 3 tbsp. cream cheese
- 6 square egg roll wrappers

Directions:
1. Place baking pan in position 2. Lightly spray fryer basket with cooking spray.
2. Heat a large skillet over med-high heat. Add beef, garlic powder, onion powder, salt and pepper. Stir to combine.
3. Add in bell pepper and onion and cook, stirring occasionally, until beef is no longer pink and vegetables are tender, about 6-8 minutes.
4. Remove from heat and drain fat. Add provolone and cream cheese and stir until melted and combined. Transfer to a large bowl.
5. Lay egg roll wrappers, one at a time, on a dry work surface. Spoon about 1/3 cup mixture in a row just below the center of the wrapper. Moisten edges with water. Fold the sides in towards the middle and roll up around filling.
6. Place egg rolls, seam side down in fryer basket. Spray lightly with cooking spray. Place the basket in the oven and set to air fry on 400°F for 10 minutes. Cook until golden brown, turning over halfway through cooking time. Serve immediately.
Nutrition Info: Calories 238, Total Fat 10g, Saturated Fat 5g, Total Carbs 21g, Net Carbs 20g, Protein 16g, Sugar 1g, Fiber 1g, Sodium 412mg, Potassium 206mg, Phosphorus 160mg

316.Turmeric Mushroom(1)

Servings: 4
Cooking Time: 20 Minutes

Ingredients:
- 1 lb. brown mushrooms
- 4 garlic cloves; minced
- ¼ tsp. cinnamon powder
- 1 tsp. olive oil
- ½ tsp. turmeric powder
- Salt and black pepper to taste.

Directions:
1. In a bowl, combine all the ingredients and toss.
2. Put the mushrooms in your air fryer's basket and cook at 370°F for 15 minutes
3. Divide the mix between plates and serve as a side dish.

Nutrition Info: Calories: 208; Fat: 7g; Fiber: 3g; Carbs: 5g; Protein: 7g

317.Garlic Roasted Asparagus

Servings: 4
Cooking Time: 10 Minutes
Ingredients:
- 1 pound (454 g) asparagus, woody ends trimmed
- 2 tablespoons olive oil
- 1 tablespoon balsamic vinegar
- 2 teaspoons minced garlic
- Salt and freshly ground black pepper, to taste

Directions:
1. In a large shallow bowl, toss the asparagus with the olive oil, balsamic vinegar, garlic, salt, and pepper until thoroughly coated. Put the asparagus in the air fryer basket.
2. Put the air fryer basket on the baking pan and slide into Rack Position 2, select Roast, set temperature to 400ºF (205ºC), and set time to 10 minutes.
3. Flip the asparagus with tongs halfway through the cooking time.
4. When cooking is complete, the asparagus should be crispy. Remove from the oven and serve warm.

318.Parmesan Zucchini Chips

Servings: 4
Cooking Time: 20 Minutes
Ingredients:
- 1 oz. pork rinds.
- ½ cup grated Parmesan cheese.
- 2 medium zucchini
- 1 large egg.

Directions:
1. Slice zucchini in ¼-inch-thick slices. Place between two layers of paper towels or a clean kitchen towel for 30 minutes to remove excess moisture

2. Place pork rinds into food processor and pulse until finely ground. Pour into medium bowl and mix with Parmesan
3. Beat egg in a small bowl.
4. Dip zucchini slices in egg and then in pork rind mixture, coating as completely as possible. Carefully place each slice into the air fryer basket in a single layer, working in batches as necessary.
5. Adjust temperature to 320 Degrees F and set the timer for 10 minutes. Flip chips halfway through the cooking time. Serve warm.

Nutrition Info: Calories: 121; Protein: 9.9g; Fiber: 0.6g; Fat: 6.7g; Carbs: 3.8g

319.Turmeric Mushroom(2)

Servings: 4
Cooking Time: 8 Minutes
Ingredients:
- 1 lb. brown mushrooms
- 4 garlic cloves; minced
- ¼ tsp. cinnamon powder
- 1 tsp. olive oil
- ½ tsp. turmeric powder
- Salt and black pepper to taste.

Directions:
1. In a bowl, combine all the ingredients and toss.
2. Put the mushrooms in your air fryer's basket and cook at 370°F for 15 minutes
3. Divide the mix between plates and serve as a side dish.

Nutrition Info: Calories: 208; Fat: 7g; Fiber: 3g; Carbs: 5g; Protein: 7g

320.Sweet Coconut Shrimp

Servings: 4
Cooking Time: 25 Minutes
Ingredients:
- 1 lb jumbo shrimp, peeled and deveined
- ¾ cup shredded coconut
- 1 tbsp maple syrup
- ½ cup breadcrumbs
- ⅓ cup cornstarch
- ½ cup milk

Directions:
1. Pour the cornstarch in a zipper bag and add in the shrimp. Seal the bag and shake vigorously to coat. In a bowl, mix the syrup with milk. In a separate bowl, combine the breadcrumbs and coconut. Open the zipper bag and remove the shrimp while shaking off excess starch.
2. Dip shrimp in the milk mixture and then in the crumbs, pressing loosely to trap enough crumbs and coconut. Place the coated shrimp in the basket

without overcrowding. Select AirFry function, adjust the temperature to 360 F, and press Start. Cook for 12 minutes until crispy.

321.Potato Chips With Creamy Lemon Dip

Servings: 3
Cooking Time: 25 Minutes
Ingredients:
- 3 large potatoes
- 1 cup sour cream
- 2 scallions, white part minced
- 3 tbsp olive oil.
- ½ tsp lemon juice
- salt and black pepper

Directions:
1. Preheat Breville on AirFry function to 350 F. Cut the potatoes into thin slices; do not peel them. Brush them with olive oil and season with salt and pepper. Arrange on the frying basket.
2. Press Start on the oven and cook for 20-25 minutes. Season with salt and pepper. To prepare the dip, mix together the sour cream, olive oil, scallions, lemon juice, salt, and pepper.

322.Buttered Corn

Servings: 2
Cooking Time: 20 Minutes
Ingredients:
- 2 corn on the cob
- Salt and freshly ground black pepper, as needed
- 2 tablespoons butter, softened and divided

Directions:
1. Sprinkle the cobs evenly with salt and black pepper.
2. Then, rub with 1 tablespoon of butter.
3. With 1 piece of foil, wrap each cob.
4. Press "Power Button" of Air Fry Oven and turn the dial to select the "Air Fry" mode.
5. Press the Time button and again turn the dial to set the cooking time to 20 minutes.
6. Now push the Temp button and rotate the dial to set the temperature at 320 degrees F.
7. Press "Start/Pause" button to start.
8. When the unit beeps to show that it is preheated, open the lid.
9. Arrange the cobs in "Air Fry Basket" and insert in the oven.
10. Serve warm.
Nutrition Info: Calories 186 Total Fat 12.2 g Saturated Fat 7.4 g Cholesterol 31 mg Sodium 163 mg Total Carbs 20.1 g Fiber 2.5 g Sugar 3.2g Protein 2.9 g

323.Baked Sweet Potatoes

Servings: 6
Cooking Time: 35 Minutes
Ingredients:
- 4 large sweet potatoes, peel and cut into cubes
- 8 sage leaves
- 1 tsp honey
- 2 tsp vinegar
- 1/2 tsp paprika
- 2 tbsp olive oil
- 1/2 tsp sea salt

Directions:
1. Fit the oven with the rack in position
2. Add sweet potato, oil, sage, and salt in a baking dish and mix well.
3. Set to bake at 375 F for 40 minutes. After 5 minutes place the baking dish in the preheated oven.
4. Transfer roasted sweet potatoes into the large bowl and toss with honey, vinegar, and paprika.
5. Serve and enjoy.
Nutrition Info: Calories 92 Fat 5.1 g Carbohydrates 12 g Sugar 1.2 g Protein 0.8 g Cholesterol 0 mg

324.Baked Cauliflower & Tomatoes

Servings: 4
Cooking Time: 20 Minutes
Ingredients:
- 4 cups cauliflower florets
- 1 tbsp capers, drained
- 3 tbsp olive oil
- 1/2 cup cherry tomatoes, halved
- 2 tbsp fresh parsley, chopped
- 2 garlic cloves, sliced
- Pepper
- Salt

Directions:
1. Fit the oven with the rack in position
2. In a bowl, toss together cherry tomatoes, cauliflower, oil, garlic, capers, pepper, and salt and spread in baking pan.
3. Set to bake at 450 F for 25 minutes. After 5 minutes place the baking pan in the preheated oven.
4. Garnish with parsley and serve.
Nutrition Info: Calories 123 Fat 10.7 g Carbohydrates 6.9 g Sugar 3 g Protein 2.4 g Cholesterol 0 mg

325.Baked Artichoke Hearts

Servings: 6
Cooking Time: 25 Minutes
Ingredients:
- 15 oz frozen artichoke hearts, defrosted
- 1 tbsp olive oil

- Pepper
- Salt

Directions:
1. Fit the oven with the rack in position
2. Arrange artichoke hearts in baking pan and drizzle with olive oil. Season with pepper and salt.
3. Set to bake at 400 F for 30 minutes. After 5 minutes place the baking pan in the preheated oven.
4. Serve and enjoy.

Nutrition Info: Calories 53 Fat 2.4 g Carbohydrates 7.5 g Sugar 0.7 g Protein 2.3 g Cholesterol 0 mg

326.Garlicky Mushroom Spaghetti

Servings: 4
Cooking Time: 20 Minutes
Ingredients:
- ½ lb white button mushrooms, sliced
- 1 tsp butter, softened
- 2 garlic cloves, chopped
- 12 oz spaghetti, cooked
- 14 oz mushroom sauce
- Salt and black pepper to taste

Directions:
1. Preheat Breville on AirFry function to 400 F. In a round baking dish, mix the mushrooms, butter, garlic, salt, and pepper. Press Start and cook for 10-12 minutes. Heat the mushroom sauce a pan over medium heat and stir in the mushrooms Pour over cooked spaghetti and serve.

327.Browned Ricotta With Capers And Lemon

Servings: 4 To 6
Cooking Time: 8 Minutes
Ingredients:
- 1½ cups whole milk ricotta cheese
- 2 tablespoons extra-virgin olive oil
- 2 tablespoons capers, rinsed
- Zest of 1 lemon, plus more for garnish
- 1 teaspoon finely chopped fresh rosemary
- Pinch crushed red pepper flakes
- Salt and freshly ground black pepper, to taste
- 1 tablespoon grated Parmesan cheese
- In a mixing bowl, stir together the ricotta cheese, olive oil, capers, lemon zest, rosemary, red pepper flakes, salt, and pepper until well combined.

Directions:
1. Spread the mixture evenly in the baking pan.
2. Slide the baking pan into Rack Position 2, select Air Fry, set temperature to 380ºF (193ºC), and set time to 8 minutes.
3. When cooking is complete, the top should be nicely browned. Remove from the oven and top with

a sprinkle of grated Parmesan cheese. Garnish with the lemon zest and serve warm.

328.Mexican Rice

Servings: 8
Cooking Time: 4 Minutes
Ingredients:
- ½ cup chopped fresh cilantro
- 1 cup of long grain rice
- 1 cup of vegetable broth
- ¼ cup of hot green sauce
- ½ avocado, salt, peeled and chopped
- Salt and freshly ground black pepper, to taste

Directions:
1. Put the rice in the instant pot, add the broth, stir, cover and cook for 4 minutes.
2. Release the pressure naturally for 10 minutes, uncover the Instant Pot, fluff it with a fork and transfer it to a bowl.
3. In a food processor, mix the avocado with the hot sauce and the cilantro and mash until smooth.
4. Pour over the rice, mix well, add salt and pepper, stir again, divide between the plates and serve.

Nutrition Info: Calories: 100, Fat: 2, Fiber: 1, Carbohydrate: 18, Proteins: 2

329.Dill Pickles With Parmesan

Servings: 4
Cooking Time: 35 Minutes
Ingredients:
- 3 cups dill pickles, sliced, drained
- 2 eggs
- 2 tsp water
- 1 cup grated Parmesan cheese
- 1 ½ cups breadcrumbs, smooth
- Black pepper to taste

Directions:
1. Preheat on Air Fry function to 400 F. In a bowl, add the breadcrumbs and black pepper and mix well. In another bowl, crack the eggs and beat with the water. Add the Parmesan cheese to a separate bowl.
2. Pull out the fryer basket and spray it lightly with cooking spray. Dredge the pickle slices it in the egg mixture, then in breadcrumbs and then in cheese. Place them in the basket without overlapping and fit in the baking tray. Cook for 4 minutes. Turn them and cook for further for 5 minutes until crispy. Serve with cheese dip.

330.Homemade Cheddar Biscuits

Servings: 8
Cooking Time: 35 Minutes

Ingredients:
- ½ cup + 1 tbsp butter
- 2 tbsp sugar
- 3 cups flour
- 1 ⅓ cups buttermilk
- ½ cup cheddar cheese, grated

Directions:
1. Preheat on Bake function to 380 F. Lay a parchment paper on a baking plate. In a bowl, mix sugar, flour, ½ cup of butter, half of the cheddar cheese, and buttermilk to form a batter. Make 8 balls from the batter and roll in flour.
2. Place the balls in your Air Fryer baking tray and flatten into biscuit shapes. Sprinkle the remaining cheddar cheese and remaining butter on top. Cook for 30 minutes, tossing every 10 minutes. Serve.

331.Bacon Wrapped Asparagus

Servings: 4
Cooking Time: 4
Ingredients:
- 20 spears asparagus
- 4 bacon slices
- 1 tbsp olive oil
- 1 tbsp sesame oil
- 1 tbsp brown sugar
- 1 garlic clove, crushed

Directions:
1. Preheat on Air Fry function to 380 F. In a bowl, mix the oils, sugar, and crushed garlic. Separate the asparagus into 4 bunches (5 spears in 1 bunch) and wrap each bunch with a bacon slice. Coat the bunches with the oil mixture. Place them in your Air Fryer basket and fit in the baking tray. Cook for 8 minutes, shaling once. Serve warm.

332.Charred Green Beans With Sesame Seeds

Servings: 4
Cooking Time: 8 Minutes
Ingredients:
- 1 tablespoon reduced-sodium soy sauce or tamari
- ½ tablespoon Sriracha sauce
- 4 teaspoons toasted sesame oil, divided
- 12 ounces (340 g) trimmed green beans
- ½ tablespoon toasted sesame seeds

Directions:
1. Whisk together the soy sauce, Sriracha sauce, and 1 teaspoon of sesame oil in a small bowl until smooth. Set aside.
2. Toss the green beans with the remaining sesame oil in a large bowl until evenly coated.

3. Place the green beans in the air fryer basket in a single layer.
4. Put the air fryer basket on the baking pan and slide into Rack Position 2, select Air Fry, set temperature to 375ºF (190ºC), and set time to 8 minutes.
5. Stir the green beans halfway through the cooking time.
6. When cooking is complete, the green beans should be lightly charred and tender. Remove from the oven to a platter. Pour the prepared sauce over the top of green beans and toss well. Serve sprinkled with the toasted sesame seeds.

333.Cheddar Cheese Cauliflower Casserole

Servings: 8
Cooking Time: 35 Minutes
Ingredients:
- 4 cups cauliflower florets
- 1 1/2 cups cheddar cheese, shredded
- 1 cup sour cream
- 4 bacon slices, cooked and crumbled
- 3 green onions, chopped

Directions:
1. Fit the oven with the rack in position
2. Boil water in a large pot. Add cauliflower in boiling water and cook for 8-10 minutes or until tender. Drain well.
3. Transfer cauliflower in a large bowl.
4. Add half bacon, half green onion, 1 cup cheese, and sour cream in cauliflower bowl and mix well.
5. Transfer mixture into a greased baking dish and sprinkle with remaining cheese.
6. Set to bake at 350 F for 30 minutes. After 5 minutes place the baking dish in the preheated oven.
7. Garnish with remaining green onion and bacon.
8. Serve and enjoy.

Nutrition Info: Calories 213 Fat 17.1 g Carbohydrates 4.7 g Sugar 1.5 g Protein 10.8 g Cholesterol 45 mg

334.Garlic Lemon Roasted Chicken

Servings: 4
Cooking Time: 60 Minutes
Ingredients:
- 1 (3 ½ pounds) whole chicken
- 2 tbsp olive oil
- Salt and black pepper to taste
- 1 lemon, cut into quarters
- 5 garlic cloves

Directions:
1. Preheat on Air Fry function to 360 F. Brush the chicken with olive oil and season with salt and

pepper. Stuff with lemon and garlic cloves into the cavity.

2.   Place the chicken breast-side down onto the Air Fryer basket. Tuck the legs and wings tips under. Fit in the baking tray and cook for 45 minutes at 350 F on Bake function. Let rest for 5-6 minutes, then carve and serve.

335.Avocado Fries

Servings: 4
Cooking Time: 20 Minutes
Ingredients:
- 1 oz. pork rinds, finely ground
- 2 medium avocados

Directions:
1.   Cut each avocado in half. Remove the pit. Carefully remove the peel and then slice the flesh into ¼-inch-thick slices.
2.   Place the pork rinds into a medium bowl and press each piece of avocado into the pork rinds to coat completely. Place the avocado pieces into the air fryer basket. Adjust the temperature to 350 Degrees F and set the timer for 5 minutes. Serve immediately
Nutrition Info: Calories: 153; Protein: 4g; Fiber: 6g; Fat: 19g; Carbs: 9g

336.Balsamic-glazed Carrots

Servings: 3
Cooking Time: 18 Minutes
Ingredients:
- 3 medium-size carrots, cut into 2-inch × ½-inch sticks
- 1 tablespoon orange juice
- 2 teaspoons balsamic vinegar
- 1 teaspoon maple syrup
- 1 teaspoon avocado oil
- ½ teaspoon dried rosemary
- ¼ teaspoon sea salt
- ¼ teaspoon lemon zest

Directions:
1.   Put the carrots in the baking pan and sprinkle with the orange juice, balsamic vinegar, maple syrup, avocado oil, rosemary, sea salt, finished by the lemon zest. Toss well.
2.   Slide the baking pan into Rack Position 2, select Roast, set temperature to 392ºF (200ºC), and set time to 18 minutes.
3.   Stir the carrots several times during the cooking process.
4.   When cooking is complete, the carrots should be nicely glazed and tender. Remove from the oven and serve hot.

337.Shrimp With Spices

Servings: 3
Cooking Time: 15 Minutes
Ingredients:
- ½ pound shrimp, deveined
- ½ tsp Cajun seasoning
- Salt and black pepper to taste
- 1 tbsp olive oil
- ¼ tsp paprika

Directions:
1.   Preheat on Air Fry function to 390 F. In a bowl, mix paprika, salt, pepper, olive oil, and Cajun seasoning. Add in the shrimp and toss to coat. Transfer the prepared shrimp to the AirFryer basket and fit in the baking tray. Cook for 10-12 minutes, flipping halfway through.

338.Grilled Sandwich With Ham & Cheese

Servings: 2
Cooking Time: 15 Minutes
Ingredients:
- 4 bread slices
- ¼ cup butter
- 2 ham slices
- 2 mozzarella cheese slices

Directions:
1.   Preheat Breville on AirFry function to 360 degrees F. Place 2 bread slices on a flat surface. Spread butter on the exposed surfaces. Lay cheese and ham on two of the slices.
2.   Cover with the other 2 slices to form sandwiches. Place the sandwiches in the frying basket. Select Bake function, adjust the temperature to 380 F, and press Start. Cook for 5 minutes.

339.Drunken Peas

Servings: 4
Cooking Time: 7 Minutes
Ingredients:
- 1 pound fresh peas
- 4 ounces smoked pancetta, chopped
- 1 green onion, sliced
- ¼ cup beer
- 1 tablespoon fresh mint, chopped
- 1 tablespoon butter
- Salt and ground black pepper, to taste
- 2 cups water

Directions:
1.   Place the water in the instant jug, place the steam basket and set aside. In a heat-resistant skillet, mix the bacon with half the onion and spread over the bottom.

2. Heat on the stove over medium-high heat for 3 minutes, add beer, peas and salt, stir and remove from heat. Cover this pan with aluminum foil, place it in the steam basket, cover the Instant Pot and cook for 1 minute in the Manual setting.
3. Relieve the pressure, uncover the pan, add salt, pepper, mint and butter, mix, divide between the dishes and serve with the rest of the onion sprinkled on top.
Nutrition Info: Calories: 134, Fat: 2, Fiber: 2.5, Carbohydrate: 10, Proteins: 4.3

340.Lemon Parmesan And Peas Risotto

Servings: 6
Cooking Time: 17 Minutes
Ingredients:
- 2 tablespoons butter
- 1½ cup rice
- 1 yellow onion, peeled and chopped
- 1 tablespoon extra-virgin olive oil
- 1 teaspoon lemon zest, grated
- 3½ cups chicken stock
- 2 tablespoons lemon juice
- 2 tablespoons parsley, diced
- 2 tablespoons Parmesan cheese, finely grated
- Salt and ground black pepper, to taste
- 1½ cup peas

Directions:
1. Put the Instant Pot in the sauté mode, add 1 tablespoon of butter and oil and heat them. Add the onion, mix and cook for 5 minutes.
2. Add the rice, mix and cook for another 3 minutes. Add 3 cups of broth and lemon juice, mix, cover and cook for 5 minutes on rice.
3. Release the pressure, put the Instant Pot in manual mode, add the peas and the rest of the broth, stir and cook for 2 minutes.
4. Add the cheese, parsley, remaining butter, lemon zest, salt and pepper to taste and mix. Divide between plates and serve.
Nutrition Info: Calories: 140, Fat: 1.5, Fiber: 1, Carbohydrate: 27, Proteins: 5

341.Feta Butterbeans With Crispy Bacon

Servings: 2
Cooking Time: 10 Minutes
Ingredients:
- 1 (14 oz) can butter beans
- 1 tbsp chives
- 3 ½ oz feta, crumbled
- Black pepper to taste
- 1 tsp olive oil
- 3 ½ oz bacon, sliced

Directions:
1. Preheat on Air Fry function to 340 F. Blend beans, olive oil, and pepper in a blender. Arrange bacon slices on your Air fryer basket. Sprinkle chives on top and fit in the baking pan. Cook for 12 minutes. Add feta cheese to the bean mixture and stir. Serve bacon with the dip.

342.Parmesan Cabbage Wedges

Servings: 4
Cooking Time: 30 Minutes
Ingredients:
- ½ head cabbage, cut into wedges
- 4 tbsp butter, melted
- 2 cup Parmesan cheese, grated
- Salt and black pepper to taste
- 1 tsp smoked paprika

Directions:
1. Preheat Breville on AirFry function to 330 F. Line a baking sheet with parchment paper. Brush the cabbage wedges with butter and season with salt and pepper.
2. Coat the cabbage with the Parmesan cheese and arrange on the baking sheet; sprinkle with paprika. Press Start and cook for 15 minutes. Flip the wedges over and cook for an additional 10 minutes. Serve with yogurt dip.

FISH & SEAFOOD RECIPES

343.Breaded Seafood

Servings: 4
Cooking Time: 15 Minutes
Ingredients:
- 1 lb scallops, mussels, fish fillets, prawns, shrimp
- 2 eggs, lightly beaten
- Salt and black pepper to taste
- 1 cup breadcrumbs mixed with zest of 1 lemon

Directions:
1. Dip the seafood pieces into the eggs and season with salt and black pepper. Coat in the crumbs and spray with cooking spray. Arrange them on the frying basket and press Start. Cook for 10 minutes at 400 F on AirFry function. Serve with lemon wedges.

344.Delightful Catfish Fillets

Servings: 4
Cooking Time: 25 Minutes
Ingredients:
- 4 catfish fillets
- ¼ cup seasoned fish fry
- 1 tbsp olive oil
- 1 tbsp parsley, chopped

Directions:
1. Add seasoned fish fry and catfish fillets in a large Ziploc bag and massage well to coat. Place the fillets in your Air Fryer basket and fit in the baking tray; cook for 10 minutes at 360 F on Air Fry function. Flip the fish and cook for 2-3 more minutes. Top with parsley and serve.

345.Cheesy Tilapia Fillets

Servings: 4
Cooking Time: 15 Minutes
Ingredients:
- ¾ cup grated Parmesan cheese
- 1 tbsp olive oil
- 2 tsp paprika
- 1 tbsp chopped parsley
- ¼ tsp garlic powder
- 4 tilapia fillets

Directions:
1. Preheat on Air Fry function to 350 F. Mix parsley, Parmesan cheese, garlic, and paprika in a bowl. Brush the olive oil over the fillets and then coat with the Parmesan mixture. Place the tilapia onto a lined baking sheet and cook for 8-10 minutes, turning once. Serve.

346.Roasted Nicoise Salad

Servings: 4
Cooking Time: 15 Minutes
Ingredients:
- 10 ounces (283 g) small red potatoes, quartered
- 8 tablespoons extra-virgin olive oil, divided
- 1 teaspoon kosher salt, divided
- ½ pound (227 g) green beans, trimmed
- 1 pint cherry tomatoes
- 1 teaspoon Dijon mustard
- 3 tablespoons red wine vinegar
- Freshly ground black pepper, to taste
- 1 (9-ounce / 255-g) bag spring greens, washed and dried if needed
- 2 (5-ounce / 142-g) cans oil-packed tuna, drained
- 2 hard-cooked eggs, peeled and quartered
- $^1/_3$ cup kalamata olives, pitted

Directions:
1. In a large bowl, drizzle the potatoes with 1 tablespoon of olive oil and season with ¼ teaspoon of kosher salt. Transfer to the baking pan.
2. Slide the baking pan into Rack Position 2, select Roast, set temperature to 375ºF (190ºC), and set time to 15 minutes.
3. Meanwhile, in a mixing bowl, toss the green beans and cherry tomatoes with 1 tablespoon of olive oil and ¼ teaspoon of kosher salt until evenly coated.
4. After 10 minutes, remove the pan and fold in the green beans and cherry tomatoes. Return the pan to the oven and continue cooking.
5. Meanwhile, make the vinaigrette by whisking together the remaining 6 tablespoons of olive oil, mustard, vinegar, the remaining ½ teaspoon of kosher salt, and black pepper in a small bowl. Set aside.
6. When done, remove from the oven. Allow the vegetables to cool for 5 minutes.
7. Spread out the spring greens on a plate and spoon the tuna into the center of the greens. Arrange the potatoes, green beans, cheery tomatoes, and eggs around the tuna. Serve drizzled with the vinaigrette and scattered with the olives.

347.Spicy Catfish

Servings: 4
Cooking Time: 15 Minutes
Ingredients:
- 1 lb catfish fillets, cut 1/2-inch thick
- 1 tsp crushed red pepper
- 2 tsp onion powder
- 1 tbsp dried oregano, crushed

- 1/2 tsp ground cumin
- 1/2 tsp chili powder
- Pepper
- Salt

Directions:
1. Fit the oven with the rack in position
2. In a small bowl, mix cumin, chili powder, crushed red pepper, onion powder, oregano, pepper, and salt.
3. Rub fish fillets with the spice mixture and place in baking dish.
4. Set to bake at 350 F for 20 minutes. After 5 minutes place the baking dish in the preheated oven.
5. Serve and enjoy.

Nutrition Info: Calories 164 Fat 8.9 g Carbohydrates 2.3 g Sugar 0.6 g Protein 18 g Cholesterol 53 mg

348.Sweet & Spicy Lime Salmon

Servings: 6
Cooking Time: 15 Minutes
Ingredients:
- 1 1/2 lbs salmon fillets
- 3 tbsp brown sugar
- 2 tbsp fresh lime juice
- 1/3 cup olive oil
- 1/2 tsp red pepper flakes
- 2 garlic cloves, minced
- Pepper
- Salt

Directions:
1. Fit the oven with the rack in position
2. Place salmon on a prepared baking sheet and season with pepper and salt.
3. In a small bowl, whisk oil, red pepper flakes, garlic, brown sugar, and lime juice.
4. Pour oil mixture over salmon.
5. Set to bake at 350 F for 20 minutes. After 5 minutes place the baking dish in the preheated oven.
6. Serve and enjoy.

Nutrition Info: Calories 269 Fat 18.3 g Carbohydrates 6.1 g Sugar 4.7 g Protein 22.2 g Cholesterol 50 mg

349.Crab Cakes

Servings: 4
Cooking Time: 10 Minutes
Ingredients:
- 8 ounces jumbo lump crabmeat
- 1 tablespoon Old Bay Seasoning
- ⅓ cup bread crumbs
- ¼ cup diced red bell pepper
- ¼ cup diced green bell pepper
- 1 egg

- ¼ cup mayonnaise
- Juice of ½ lemon
- 1 teaspoon flour
- Cooking oil

Directions:
1. Preparing the Ingredients. In a large bowl, combine the crabmeat, Old Bay Seasoning, bread crumbs, red bell pepper, green bell pepper, egg, mayo, and lemon juice. Mix gently to combine.
2. Form the mixture into 4 patties. Sprinkle ¼ teaspoon of flour on top of each patty.
3. Air Frying. Place the crab cakes in the air fryer oven. Spray them with cooking oil. Cook for 10 minutes.
4. Serve.

350.Tomato Garlic Shrimp

Servings: 4
Cooking Time: 25 Minutes
Ingredients:
- 1 lb shrimp, peeled
- 1 tbsp garlic, sliced
- 2 cups cherry tomatoes
- 1 tbsp olive oil
- Pepper
- Salt

Directions:
1. Fit the oven with the rack in position
2. Add shrimp, oil, garlic, tomatoes, pepper, and salt into the large bowl and toss well.
3. Transfer shrimp mixture into the baking dish.
4. Set to bake at 400 F for 30 minutes. After 5 minutes place the baking dish in the preheated oven.
5. Serve and enjoy.

Nutrition Info: Calories 184 Fat 5.6 g Carbohydrates 5.9 g Sugar 2.4 g Protein 26.8 gCholesterol 239 mg

351.Salmon & Caper Cakes

Servings: 2
Cooking Time: 15 Minutes + Chilling Time
Ingredients:
- 8 oz salmon, cooked
- 1 ½ oz potatoes, mashed
- A handful of capers
- 1 tbsp fresh parsley, chopped
- Zest of 1 lemon
- 1 ¾ oz plain flour

Directions:
1. Carefully flake the salmon. In a bowl, mix the salmon, zest, capers, dill, and mashed potatoes. Form small cakes from the mixture and dust them with flour; refrigerate for 60 minutes. Preheat Breville to

350 F. Press Start and cook the cakes for 10 minutes on AirFry function. Serve chilled.

352.Thyme Rosemary Shrimp

Servings: 4
Cooking Time: 10 Minutes
Ingredients:
- 1 lb shrimp, peeled and deveined
- 1/2 tbsp fresh rosemary, chopped
- 1 tbsp olive oil
- 2 garlic cloves, minced
- 1/2 tbsp fresh thyme, chopped
- Pepper
- Salt

Directions:
1. Fit the oven with the rack in position
2. Add shrimp and remaining ingredients in a large bowl and toss well.
3. Pour shrimp mixture into the baking dish.
4. Set to bake at 400 F for 15 minutes. After 5 minutes place the baking dish in the preheated oven.
5. Serve and enjoy.
Nutrition Info: Calories 169 Fat 5.5 g Carbohydrates 2.7 g Sugar 0 g Protein 26 g Cholesterol 239 mg

353.Air-fried Scallops

Servings: 2
Cooking Time: 12 Minutes
Ingredients:
- $^1/_3$ cup shallots, chopped
- 1½ tablespoons olive oil
- 1½ tablespoons coconut aminos
- 1 tablespoon Mediterranean seasoning mix
- ½ tablespoon balsamic vinegar
- ½ teaspoon ginger, grated
- 1 clove garlic, chopped
- 1 pound (454 g) scallops, cleanedCooking spray
- Belgian endive, for garnish

Directions:
1. Place all the ingredients except the scallops and Belgian endive in a small skillet over medium heat and stir to combine. Let this mixture simmer for about 2 minutes.
2. Remove the mixture from the skillet to a large bowl and set aside to cool.
3. Add the scallops, coating them all over, then transfer to the refrigerator to marinate for at least 2 hours.
4. When ready, place the scallops in the air fryer basket in a single layer and spray with cooking spray.
5. Put the air fryer basket on the baking pan and slide into Rack Position 2, select Air Fry, set

temperature to 345ºF (174ºC), and set time to 10 minutes.
6. Flip the scallops halfway through the cooking time.
7. When cooking is complete, the scallops should be tender and opaque. Remove from the oven and serve garnished with the Belgian endive.

354.Sweet Cajun Salmon

Servings: 1
Cooking Time: 10 Minutes
Ingredients:
- 1 salmon fillet
- ¼ tsp brown sugar
- Juice of ½ lemon
- 1 tbsp cajun seasoning
- 2 lemon wedges
- 1 tbsp chopped parsley

Directions:
1. Preheat on Bake function to 350 F. Combine sugar and lemon juice; coat the salmon with this mixture. Coat with the Cajun seasoning as well. Place a parchment paper on a baking tray and cook the fish in your for 10 minutes. Serve with lemon wedges and parsley.

355.Air Fryer Spicy Shrimp

Servings: 4
Cooking Time: 6 Minutes
Ingredients:
- 1 lb shrimp, peeled and deveined
- 1/4 tsp chili powder
- 1 tsp dried oregano
- 1 tsp garlic powder
- 1 tsp onion powder
- 2 tsp paprika
- 1/4 tsp cayenne
- 2 tbsp olive oil
- Pepper
- Salt

Directions:
1. Fit the oven with the rack in position 2.
2. In a bowl, toss shrimp with remaining ingredients.
3. Add shrimp to the air fryer basket then place an air fryer basket in the baking pan.
4. Place a baking pan on the oven rack. Set to air fry at 400 F for 6 minutes.
5. Serve and enjoy.
Nutrition Info: Calories 204 Fat 9.2 g Carbohydrates 3.7 g Sugar 0.5 g Protein 26.2 g Cholesterol 239 mg

356.Shrimp With Smoked Paprika & Cayenne Pepper

Servings: 3
Cooking Time: 10 Minutes
Ingredients:
- 6 oz tiger shrimp, 12 to 16 pieces
- 1 tbsp olive oil
- ½ a tbsp old bay seasoning
- ¼ a tbsp cayenne pepper
- ¼ a tbsp smoked paprika
- A pinch of sea salt

Directions:
1. Preheat on Air Fry function to 380 F. Mix olive oil, old bay seasoning, cayenne pepper, smoked paprika, and sea salt in a large bowl. Add in the shrimp and toss to coat. Place the shrimp in the frying basket and fit in the baking tray; cook for 6-7 minutes, sahing once. Serve.

357.Fish Tacos

Servings: 6
Cooking Time: 10 To 15 Minutes
Ingredients:
- 1 tablespoon avocado oil
- 1 tablespoon Cajun seasoning
- 4 (5 to 6 ounce / 142 to 170 g) tilapia fillets
- 1 (14-ounce / 397-g) package coleslaw mix
- 12 corn tortillas
- 2 limes, cut into wedges

Directions:
1. Line the baking pan with parchment paper.
2. In a shallow bowl, stir together the avocado oil and Cajun seasoning to make a marinade. Place the tilapia fillets into the bowl, turning to coat evenly.
3. Put the fillets in the baking pan in a single layer.
4. Put the air fryer basket on the baking pan and slide into Rack Position 2, select Air Fry, set temperature to 375ºF (190ºC), and set time to 10 minutes.
5. When cooked, the fish should be flaky. If necessary, continue cooking for 5 minutes more. Remove the fish from the oven to a plate.
6. Assemble the tacos: Spoon some of the coleslaw mix into each tortilla and top each with $1/3$ of a tilapia fillet. Squeeze some lime juice over the top of each taco and serve immediately.

358.Spicy Halibut

Servings: 4
Cooking Time: 12 Minutes
Ingredients:
- 1 lb halibut fillets
- 1/2 tsp chili powder
- 1/2 tsp smoked paprika
- 1/4 cup olive oil
- 1/4 tsp garlic powder
- Pepper
- Salt

Directions:
1. Fit the oven with the rack in position
2. Place halibut fillets in a baking dish.
3. In a small bowl, mix oil, garlic powder, paprika, pepper, chili powder, and salt.
4. Brush fish fillets with oil mixture.
5. Set to bake at 425 F for 17 minutes. After 5 minutes place the baking dish in the preheated oven.
6. Serve and enjoy.
Nutrition Info: Calories 236 Fat 15.3 g Carbohydrates 0.5 g Sugar 0.1 g Protein 24 g Cholesterol 36 mg

359.Maryland Crab Cakes

Servings: 6
Cooking Time: 10 Minutes
Ingredients:
- Nonstick cooking spray
- 2 eggs
- 1 cup Panko bread crumbs
- 1 stalk celery, chopped
- 3 tbsp. mayonnaise
- 1 tsp Worcestershire sauce
- ¼ cup mozzarella cheese, grated
- 1 tsp Italian seasoning
- 1 tbsp. fresh parsley, chopped
- 1 tsp pepper
- ¾ lb. lump crabmeat, drained

Directions:
1. Place baking pan in position 2 of the oven. Lightly spray the fryer basket with cooking spray.
2. In a large bowl, combine all ingredients except crab meat, mix well.
3. Fold in crab carefully so it retains some chunks. Form mixture into 12 patties.
4. Place patties in a single layer in the fryer basket. Place the basket on the baking pan.
5. Set oven to air fryer on 350°F for 10 minutes. Cook until golden brown, turning over halfway through cooking time. Serve immediately.
Nutrition Info: Calories 172, Total Fat 8g, Saturated Fat 2g, Total Carbs 14g, Net Carbs 13g, Protein 16g, Sugar 1g, Fiber 1g, Sodium 527mg, Potassium 290mg, Phosphorus 201mg

360.Fish Cakes With Mango Relish

Servings: 4
Cooking Time: 10 Minutes

Ingredients:
- 1 lb White Fish Fillets
- 3 Tbsps Ground Coconut
- 1 Ripened Mango
- ½ Tsps Chili Paste
- Tbsps Fresh Parsley
- 1 Green Onion
- 1 Lime
- 1 Tsp Salt
- 1 Egg

Directions:
1. Preparing the Ingredients. To make the relish, peel and dice the mango into cubes. Combine with a half teaspoon of chili paste, a tablespoon of parsley, and the zest and juice of half a lime.
2. In a food processor, pulse the fish until it forms a smooth texture. Place into a bowl and add the salt, egg, chopped green onion, parsley, two tablespoons of the coconut, and the remainder of the chili paste and lime zest and juice. Combine well
3. Portion the mixture into 10 equal balls and flatten them into small patties. Pour the reserved tablespoon of coconut onto a dish and roll the patties over to coat.
4. Preheat the Air fryer oven to 390 degrees
5. Air Frying. Place the fish cakes into the air fryer oven and cook for 8 minutes. They should be crisp and lightly browned when ready
6. Serve hot with mango relish

361.Crispy Fish Sticks

Servings: 8
Cooking Time: 6 Minutes
Ingredients:
- 8 ounces (227 g) fish fillets (pollock or cod), cut into ½ × 3 inches strips
- Salt, to taste (optional)
- ½ cup plain bread crumbs
- Cooking spray

Directions:
1. Season the fish strips with salt to taste, if desired.
2. Place the bread crumbs on a plate, then roll the fish in the bread crumbs until well coated. Spray all sides of the fish with cooking spray. Transfer to the air fryer basket in a single layer.
3. Put the air fryer basket on the baking pan and slide into Rack Position 2, select Air Fry, set temperature to 400ºF (205ºC), and set time to 6 minutes.
4. When cooked, the fish sticks should be golden brown and crispy. Remove from the oven to a plate and serve hot.

362.Old Bay Tilapia Fillets

Servings: 4
Cooking Time: 15 Minutes
Ingredients:
- 1 pound tilapia fillets
- 1 tbsp old bay seasoning
- 2 tbsp canola oil
- 2 tbsp lemon pepper
- Salt to taste
- 2-3 butter buds

Directions:
1. Preheat your oven to 400 F on Bake function. Drizzle tilapia fillets with canola oil. In a bowl, mix salt, lemon pepper, butter buds, and seasoning; spread on the fish. Place the fillet on the basket and fit in the baking tray. Cook for 10 minutes, flipping once until tender and crispy.

363.Old Bay Shrimp

Servings: 4
Cooking Time: 10 Minutes
Ingredients:
- 1 lb jumbo shrimp
- Salt to taste
- ¼ tsp old bay seasoning
- ⅓ tsp smoked paprika
- ¼ tsp chili powder
- 1 tbsp olive oil

Directions:
1. Preheat Breville on AirFry function to 390 F. In a bowl, add the shrimp, paprika, oil, salt, old bay seasoning, and chili powder; mix well. Place the shrimp in the oven and cook for 5 minutes.

364.Breaded Calamari With Lemon

Servings: 4
Cooking Time: 12 Minutes
Ingredients:
- 2 large eggs
- 2 garlic cloves, minced
- ½ cup cornstarch
- 1 cup bread crumbs
- 1 pound (454 g) calamari rings
- Cooking spray
- 1 lemon, sliced

Directions:
1. In a small bowl, whisk the eggs with minced garlic. Place the cornstarch and bread crumbs into separate shallow dishes.
2. Dredge the calamari rings in the cornstarch, then dip in the egg mixture, shaking off any excess, finally roll them in the bread crumbs to coat well. Let

the calamari rings sit for 10 minutes in the refrigerator.
3. Spritz the air fryer basket with cooking spray. Transfer the calamari rings to the pan.
4. Put the air fryer basket on the baking pan and slide into Rack Position 2, select Air Fry, set temperature to 390ºF (199ºC), and set time to 12 minutes.
5. Stir the calamari rings once halfway through the cooking time.
6. When cooking is complete, remove from the oven. Serve the calamari rings with the lemon slices sprinkled on top.

365.Seafood Platter

Ingredients:
- 1 large plate with assorted prepared seafood
- 3 tbsp. vinegar or lemon juice
- 2 or 3 tsp. paprika
- 1 tsp. black pepper
- 1 tsp. salt
- 3 tsp. ginger-garlic paste
- 1 cup yogurt
- 4 tsp. tandoori masala
- 2 tbsp. dry fenugreek leaves
- 1 tsp. black salt
- 1 tsp. chat masala
- 1 tsp. garam masala powder
- 1 tsp. red chili powder
- 1 tsp. salt
- 3 drops of red color

Directions:
1. Make the first marinade and soak the seafood in it for four hours. While this is happening, make the second marinade and soak the seafood in it overnight to let the flavors blend.
2. Pre heat the oven at 160 degrees Fahrenheit for 5 minutes. Place the Oregano Fingers in the fry basket and close it. Let them cook at the same temperature for another 15 minutes or so. Toss the Oregano Fingers well so that they are cooked uniformly. Serve them with mint sauce.

366.Coconut Chili Fish Curry

Servings: 4
Cooking Time: 22 Minutes
Ingredients:
- 2 tablespoons sunflower oil, divided
- 1 pound (454 g) fish, chopped
- 1 ripe tomato, pureéd
- 2 red chilies, chopped
- 1 shallot, minced
- 1 garlic clove, minced
- 1 cup coconut milk
- 1 tablespoon coriander powder
- 1 teaspoon red curry paste
- ½ teaspoon fenugreek seeds
- Salt and white pepper, to taste

Directions:
1. Coat the air fryer basket with 1 tablespoon of sunflower oil. Place the fish in the basket.
2. Put the air fryer basket on the baking pan and slide into Rack Position 2, select Air Fry, set temperature to 380ºF (193ºC), and set time to 10 minutes.
3. Flip the fish halfway through the cooking time.
4. When cooking is complete, transfer the cooked fish to the baking pan greased with the remaining 1 tablespoon of sunflower oil. Stir in the remaining ingredients.
5. Put the air fryer basket on the baking pan and slide into Rack Position 2, select Air Fry, set temperature to 350ºF (180ºC), and set time to 12 minutes.
6. When cooking is complete, they should be heated through. Cool for 5 to 8 minutes before serving.

367.Honey Glazed Salmon

Servings: 4
Cooking Time: 8 Minutes
Ingredients:
- 4 salmon fillets
- 2 tsp soy sauce
- 1 tbsp honey
- Pepper
- Salt

Directions:
1. Fit the oven with the rack in position 2.
2. Brush salmon with soy sauce and season with pepper and salt.
3. Place salmon in the air fryer basket then place an air fryer basket in the baking pan.
4. Place a baking pan on the oven rack. Set to air fry at 375 F for 8 minutes.
5. Brush salmon with honey and serve.
Nutrition Info: Calories 253 Fat 11 g Carbohydrates 4.6 g Sugar 4.4 g Protein 34.7 g Cholesterol 78 mg

368.Smoked Paprika Tiger Shrimp

Servings: 4
Cooking Time: 10 Minutes
Ingredients:
- 1 lb tiger shrimp
- 2 tbsp olive oil
- ¼ tbsp garlic powder

- 1 tbsp smoked paprika
- 2 tbsp fresh parsley, chopped
- Sea salt to taste

Directions:
1. Preheat Breville on AirFry function to 380 F. Mix garlic powder, smoked paprika, salt, parsley, and olive oil in a large bowl. Add in the shrimp and toss to coat. Place the shrimp in the frying basket press Start. Fry for 6-7 minutes. Serve with salad.

369.Fried Cod Nuggets

Servings: 4
Cooking Time: 25 Minutes
Ingredients:
- 1 ¼ lb cod fillets, cut into 4 to 6 chunks each
- ½ cup flour
- 1 egg
- 1 cup cornflakes
- 1 tbsp olive oil
- Salt and black pepper to taste

Directions:
1. Place the olive oil and cornflakes in a food processor and process until crumbed. Season the fish chunks with salt and pepper. In a bowl, beat the egg along with 1 tbsp of water. Dredge the chunks in flour first, then dip in the egg, and finally coat with cornflakes. Arrange the fish pieces on a lined sheet and cook in your on Air Fry at 350 F for 15 minutes until crispy.

370.Lemon Butter Shrimp

Servings: 4
Cooking Time: 12 Minutes
Ingredients:
- 1 1/4 lbs shrimp, peeled & deveined
- 2 tbsp fresh parsley, chopped
- 2 tbsp fresh lemon juice
- 1 tbsp garlic, minced
- 1/4 cup butter
- Pepper
- Salt

Directions:
1. Fit the oven with the rack in position
2. Add shrimp into the baking dish.
3. Melt butter in a pan over low heat. Add garlic and sauté for 30 seconds. Stir in lemon juice.
4. Pour melted butter mixture over shrimp. Season with pepper and salt.
5. Set to bake at 350 F for 17 minutes. After 5 minutes place the baking dish in the preheated oven.
6. Garnish with parsley and serve.
Nutrition Info: Calories 276 Fat 14 g Carbohydrates 3.2 g Sugar 0.2 g Protein 32.7 g Cholesterol 329 mg

371.Old Bay Seasoned Scallops

Servings: 4
Cooking Time: 4 Minutes
Ingredients:
- 1 lb sea scallops
- 1/2 tsp garlic powder
- 1/2 cup crushed crackers
- 2 tbsp butter, melted
- 1/2 tsp old bay seasoning

Directions:
1. Fit the oven with the rack in position 2.
2. In a shallow dish, mix crushed crackers, garlic powder, and old bay seasoning.
3. Add melted butter in a separate shallow dish.
4. Dip scallops in melted butter and coat with crushed crackers.
5. Place coated scallops in air fryer basket then place air fryer basket in baking pan.
6. Place a baking pan on the oven rack. Set to air fry at 390 F for 4 minutes.
7. Serve and enjoy.
Nutrition Info: Calories 167 Fat 7.4 g Carbohydrates 4.8 g Sugar 0.5 g Protein 19.5 g Cholesterol 53 mg

372.Easy Salmon Patties

Servings: 6 Patties
Cooking Time: 11 Minutes
Ingredients:
- 1 (14.75-ounce / 418-g) can Alaskan pink salmon, drained and bones removed
- ½ cup bread crumbs
- 1 egg, whisked
- 2 scallions, diced
- 1 teaspoon garlic powder
- Salt and pepper, to taste
- Cooking spray

Directions:
1. Stir together the salmon, bread crumbs, whisked egg, scallions, garlic powder, salt, and pepper in a large bowl until well incorporated.
2. Divide the salmon mixture into six equal portions and form each into a patty with your hands.
3. Arrange the salmon patties in the air fryer basket and spritz them with cooking spray.
4. Put the air fryer basket on the baking pan and slide into Rack Position 2, select Air Fry, set temperature to 400ºF (205ºC), and set time to 10 minutes.
5. Flip the patties once halfway through.
6. When cooking is complete, the patties should be golden brown and cooked through. Remove the patties from the oven and serve on a plate.

373.Prawn Momo's Recipe

Ingredients:
- 1 ½ cup all-purpose flour
- ½ tsp. salt
- 5 tbsp. water
- For filling:
- 2 cups minced prawn
- 2 tbsp. oil
- 2 tsp. ginger-garlic paste
- 2 tsp. soya sauce
- 2 tsp. vinegar

Directions:
1. Squeeze the dough and cover it with plastic wrap and set aside. Next, cook the ingredients for the filling and try to ensure that the prawn is covered well with the sauce. Roll the dough and cut it into a square.
2. Place the filling in the center. Now, wrap the dough to cover the filling and pinch the edges together. Pre heat the oven at 200° F for 5 minutes. Place the wontons in the fry basket and close it. Let them cook at the same temperature for another 20 minutes. Recommended sides are chili sauce or ketchup.

374.Herbed Scallops With Vegetables

Servings: 4
Cooking Time: 9 Minutes
Ingredients:
- 1 cup frozen peas
- 1 cup green beans
- 1 cup frozen chopped broccoli
- 2 teaspoons olive oil
- ½ teaspoon dried oregano
- ½ teaspoon dried basil
- 12 ounces (340 g) sea scallops, rinsed and patted dry

Directions:
1. Put the peas, green beans, and broccoli in a large bowl. Drizzle with the olive oil and toss to coat well. Transfer the vegetables to the air fryer basket.
2. Put the air fryer basket on the baking pan and slide into Rack Position 2, select Air Fry, set temperature to 400ºF (205ºC), and set time to 5 minutes.
3. When cooking is complete, the vegetables should be fork-tender. Transfer the vegetables to a serving bowl. Scatter with the oregano and basil and set aside.
4. Place the scallops in the basket.
5. Put the air fryer basket on the baking pan and slide into Rack Position 2, select Air Fry, set temperature to 400ºF (205ºC), and set time to 4 minutes.
6. When cooking is complete, the scallops should be firm and just opaque in the center. Remove from the oven to the bowl of vegetables and toss well. Serve warm.

375.Fired Shrimp With Mayonnaise Sauce

Servings: 4
Cooking Time: 7 Minutes
Ingredients:
- Shrimp
- 12 jumbo shrimp
- ½ teaspoon garlic salt
- ¼ teaspoon freshly cracked mixed peppercorns
- Sauce:
- 4 tablespoons mayonnaise
- 1 teaspoon grated lemon rind
- 1 teaspoon Dijon mustard
- 1 teaspoon chipotle powder
- ½ teaspoon cumin powder

Directions:
1. In a medium bowl, season the shrimp with garlic salt and cracked mixed peppercorns.
2. Place the shrimp in the air fryer basket.
3. Put the air fryer basket on the baking pan and slide into Rack Position 2, select Air Fry, set temperature to 395ºF (202ºC), and set time to 7 minutes.
4. After 5 minutes, remove from the oven and flip the shrimp. Return to the oven and continue cooking for 2 minutes more, or until they are pink and no longer opaque.
5. Meanwhile, stir together all the ingredients for the sauce in a small bowl until well mixed.
6. When cooking is complete, remove the shrimp from the oven and serve alongside the sauce.

376.Crab Cakes With Bell Peppers

Servings: 4
Cooking Time: 10 Minutes
Ingredients:
- 8 ounces (227 g) jumbo lump crab meat
- 1 egg, beaten
- Juice of ½ lemon
- $^1/_3$ cup bread crumbs
- ¼ cup diced green bell pepper
- ¼ cup diced red bell pepper
- ¼ cup mayonnaise
- 1 tablespoon Old Bay seasoning
- 1 teaspoon flour
- Cooking spray

Directions:

1. Make the crab cakes: Place all the ingredients except the flour and oil in a large bowl and stir until well incorporated.
2. Divide the crab mixture into four equal portions and shape each portion into a patty with your hands. Top each patty with a sprinkle of ¼ teaspoon of flour.
3. Arrange the crab cakes in the air fryer basket and spritz them with cooking spray.
4. Put the air fryer basket on the baking pan and slide into Rack Position 2, select Air Fry, set temperature to 375ºF (190ºC), and set time to 10 minutes.
5. Flip the crab cakes halfway through.
6. When cooking is complete, the cakes should be cooked through. Remove from the oven and divide the crab cakes among four plates and serve.

377.Shrimp And Cherry Tomato Kebabs

Servings: 4
Cooking Time: 5 Minutes
Ingredients:
- 1½ pounds (680 g) jumbo shrimp, cleaned, shelled and deveined
- 1 pound (454 g) cherry tomatoes
- 2 tablespoons butter, melted
- 1 tablespoons Sriracha sauce
- Sea salt and ground black pepper, to taste
- 1 teaspoon dried parsley flakes
- ½ teaspoon dried basil
- ½ teaspoon dried oregano
- ½ teaspoon mustard seeds
- ½ teaspoon marjoram
- Special Equipment:
- 4 to 6 wooden skewers, soaked in water for 30 minutes

Directions:
1. Put all the ingredients in a large bowl and toss to coat well.
2. Make the kebabs: Thread, alternating jumbo shrimp and cherry tomatoes, onto the wooden skewers. Place the kebabs in the air fryer basket.
3. Put the air fryer basket on the baking pan and slide into Rack Position 2, select Air Fry, set temperature to 400ºF (205ºC), and set time to 5 minutes.
4. When cooking is complete, the shrimp should be pink and the cherry tomatoes should be softened. Remove from the oven. Let the shrimp and cherry tomato kebabs cool for 5 minutes and serve hot.

378.Bacon Wrapped Shrimp

Servings: 4
Cooking Time: 5 Minutes

Ingredients:
- 1¼ pound tiger shrimp, peeled and deveined
- 1 pound bacon

Directions:
1. Preparing the Ingredients. Wrap each shrimp with a slice of bacon.
2. Refrigerate for about 20 minutes.
3. Preheat the air fryer oven to 390 degrees F.
4. Air Frying. Arrange the shrimp in the Oven rack/basket. Place the Rack on the middle-shelf of the air fryer oven. Cook for about 5-7 minutes.

379.Baked Lemon Swordfish

Servings: 2
Cooking Time: 10 Minutes
Ingredients:
- 12 oz swordfish fillets
- 1/8 tsp crushed red pepper
- 1 garlic clove, minced
- 2 tsp fresh parsley, chopped
- 3 tbsp olive oil
- 1/2 tsp lemon zest, grated
- 1/2 tsp ginger, grated

Directions:
1. Fit the oven with the rack in position
2. In a small bowl, mix 2 tbsp oil, lemon zest, red pepper, ginger, garlic, and parsley.
3. Season fish fillets with salt.
4. Heat remaining oil in a pan over medium-high heat.
5. Place fish fillets in the pan and cook until browned, about 2-3 minutes.
6. Transfer fish fillets in a baking dish.
7. Set to bake at 400 F for 15 minutes. After 5 minutes place the baking dish in the preheated oven.
8. Pour oil mixture over fish fillets and serve.
Nutrition Info: Calories 449 Fat 29.8 g Carbohydrates 1.1 g Sugar 0.1 g Protein 43.4 g Cholesterol 85 mg

380.Golden Beer-battered Cod

Servings: 4
Cooking Time: 15 Minutes
Ingredients:
- 2 eggs
- 1 cup malty beer
- 1 cup all-purpose flour
- ½ cup cornstarch
- 1 teaspoon garlic powder
- Salt and pepper, to taste
- 4 (4-ounce / 113-g) cod fillets
- Cooking spray

Directions:

1. In a shallow bowl, beat together the eggs with the beer. In another shallow bowl, thoroughly combine the flour and cornstarch. Sprinkle with the garlic powder, salt, and pepper.
2. Dredge each cod fillet in the flour mixture, then in the egg mixture. Dip each piece of fish in the flour mixture a second time.
3. Spritz the air fryer basket with cooking spray. Arrange the cod fillets in the pan in a single layer.
4. Put the air fryer basket on the baking pan and slide into Rack Position 2, select Air Fry, set temperature to 400ºF (205ºC), and set time to 15 minutes.
5. Flip the fillets halfway through the cooking time.
6. When cooking is complete, the cod should reach an internal temperature of 145ºF (63ºC) on a meat thermometer and the outside should be crispy. Let the fish cool for 5 minutes and serve.

381.Carp Flat Cakes

Ingredients:
- 2 tbsp. garam masala
- 1 lb. fileted carp
- 3 tsp ginger finely chopped
- 1-2 tbsp. fresh coriander leaves
- 2 or 3 green chilies finely chopped
- 1 ½ tbsp. lemon juice
- Salt and pepper to taste

Directions:
1. Mix the ingredients in a clean bowl and add water to it. Make sure that the paste is not too watery but is enough to apply on the sides of the carp filets.
2. Pre heat the oven at 160 degrees Fahrenheit for 5 minutes. Place the French Cuisine Galettes in the fry basket and let them cook for another 25 minutes at the same temperature. Keep rolling them over to get a uniform cook. Serve either with mint sauce or ketchup.

382.Lemon Pepper Tilapia Fillets

Servings: 4
Cooking Time: 15 Minutes
Ingredients:
- 1 lb tilapia fillets
- 1 tbsp Italian seasoning
- 2 tbsp canola oil
- 2 tbsp lemon pepper
- Salt to taste
- 2-3 butter buds

Directions:
1. Preheat your Breville oven to 400 F on Bake function. Drizzle tilapia fillets with canola oil. In a bowl, mix salt, lemon pepper, butter buds, and Italian

seasoning; spread on the fish. Place the fillet on a baking tray and press Start. Cook for 10 minutes until tender and crispy. Serve warm.

383.Spicy Lemon Garlic Tilapia

Servings: 2
Cooking Time: 15 Minutes
Ingredients:
- 4 tilapia fillets
- 1 lemon, cut into slices
- 1/2 tsp pepper
- 1/2 tsp chili powder
- 1 tsp garlic, minced
- 3 tbsp butter, melted
- 1 tbsp fresh lemon juice
- Salt

Directions:
1. Fit the oven with the rack in position
2. Place fish fillets into the baking dish.
3. Arrange lemon slices on top of fish fillets.
4. Mix together the remaining ingredients and pour over fish fillets.
5. Set to bake at 350 F for 20 minutes. After 5 minutes place the baking dish in the preheated oven.
6. Serve and enjoy.
Nutrition Info: Calories 354 Fat 19.6 g Carbohydrates 4 g Sugar 1 g Protein 42.8 g Cholesterol 156 mg

384.Baked Flounder Fillets

Servings: 2
Cooking Time: 12 Minutes
Ingredients:
- 2 flounder fillets, patted dry
- 1 egg
- ½ teaspoon Worcestershire sauce
- ¼ cup almond flour
- ¼ cup coconut flour
- ½ teaspoon coarse sea salt
- ½ teaspoon lemon pepper
- ¼ teaspoon chili powder
- Cooking spray

Directions:
1. In a shallow bowl, beat together the egg with Worcestershire sauce until well incorporated.
2. In another bowl, thoroughly combine the almond flour, coconut flour, sea salt, lemon pepper, and chili powder.
3. Dredge the fillets in the egg mixture, shaking off any excess, then roll in the flour mixture to coat well.
4. Spritz the baking pan with cooking spray. Place the fillets in the pan.

5. Slide the baking pan into Rack Position 1, select Convection Bake, set temperature to 390ºF (199ºC), and set time to 12 minutes.

6. After 7 minutes, remove from the oven and flip the fillets and spray with cooking spray. Return the pan to the oven and continue cooking for 5 minutes, or until the fish is flaky.

7. When cooking is complete, remove from the oven and serve warm.

385.Firecracker Shrimp

Servings: 4
Cooking Time: 8 Minutes
Ingredients:
- For the shrimp
- 1 pound raw shrimp, peeled and deveined
- Salt
- Pepper
- 1 egg
- ½ cup all-purpose flour
- ¾ cup panko bread crumbs
- Cooking oil
- For the firecracker sauce
- ⅓ cup sour cream
- 2 tablespoons Sriracha
- ¼ cup sweet chili sauce

Directions:
1. Preparing the Ingredients. Season the shrimp with salt and pepper to taste. In a small bowl, beat the egg. In another small bowl, place the flour. In a third small bowl, add the panko bread crumbs.

2. Spray the Oven rack/basket with cooking oil. Dip the shrimp in the flour, then the egg, and then the bread crumbs. Place the shrimp in the Oven rack/basket. It is okay to stack them. Spray the shrimp with cooking oil. Place the Rack on the middle-shelf of the air fryer oven.

3. Air Frying. Cook for 4 minutes. Open the air fryer oven and flip the shrimp. I recommend flipping individually instead of shaking to keep the breading intact. Cook for an additional 4 minutes or until crisp.

4. While the shrimp is cooking, make the firecracker sauce: In a small bowl, combine the sour cream, Sriracha, and sweet chili sauce. Mix well. Serve with the shrimp.

Nutrition Info: CALORIES: 266; CARBS:23g; FAT:6G; PROTEIN:27G; FIBER:1G

386.Tasty Lemon Pepper Basa

Servings: 4
Cooking Time: 12 Minutes
Ingredients:
- 4 basa fish fillets
- 8 tsp olive oil
- 2 tbsp fresh parsley, chopped
- 1/4 cup green onion, sliced
- 1/2 tsp garlic powder
- 1/4 tsp lemon pepper seasoning
- 4 tbsp fresh lemon juice
- Pepper
- Salt

Directions:
1. Fit the oven with the rack in position
2. Place fish fillets in a baking dish.
3. Pour remaining ingredients over fish fillets.
4. Set to bake at 425 F for 12 minutes. After 5 minutes place the baking dish in the preheated oven.
5. Serve and enjoy.

Nutrition Info: Calories 308 Fat 21.4 g Carbohydrates 5.5 g Sugar 3.4 g Protein 24.1 g Cholesterol 0 mg

387.Spicy Grilled Halibut

Servings: 4
Cooking Time: 10 Minutes
Ingredients:
- ½ cup fresh lemon juice
- 2 jalapeno peppers, seeded & chopped fine
- 4 6 oz. halibut fillets
- Nonstick cooking spray
- ¼ cup cilantro, chopped

Directions:
1. In a small bowl, combine lemon juice and chilies, mix well.
2. Place fish in a large Ziploc bag and add marinade. Toss to coat. Refrigerate 30 minutes.
3. Lightly spray the baking pan with cooking spray. Set oven to broil on 400°F for 15 minutes.
4. After 5 minutes, lay fish on the pan and place in position 2 of the oven. Cook 10 minutes, or until fish flakes easily with a fork. Turn fish over and brush with marinade halfway through cooking time.
5. Sprinkle with cilantro before serving.

Nutrition Info: Calories 328, Total Fat 24g, Saturated Fat 4g, Total Carbs 3g, Net Carbs 3g, Protein 25g, Sugar 1g, Fiber 0g, Sodium 137mg, Potassium 510mg, Phosphorus 284mg

388.Delicious Crab Cakes

Servings: 5
Cooking Time: 10 Minutes
Ingredients:
- 18 oz can crab meat, drained
- 2 1/2 tbsp mayonnaise
- 2 eggs, lightly beaten
- 1/4 cup breadcrumbs

- 1 1/2 tsp dried parsley
- 1 tbsp dried celery
- 1 tsp Old bay seasoning
- 1 1/2 tbsp Dijon mustard
- Pepper
- Salt

Directions:
1. Fit the oven with the rack in position 2.
2. Add all ingredients into the mixing bowl and mix until well combined.
3. Make patties from mixture and place in the air fryer basket then place an air fryer basket in the baking pan.
4. Place a baking pan on the oven rack. Set to air fry at 320 F for 10 minutes.
5. Serve and enjoy.

Nutrition Info: Calories 138 Fat 4.7 g Carbohydrates 7.8 g Sugar 2.7 g Protein 16.8 g Cholesterol 127 mg

389.Baked Tilapia With Garlic Aioli

Servings: 4
Cooking Time: 15 Minutes
Ingredients:
- Tilapia:
- 4 tilapia fillets
- 1 tablespoon extra-virgin olive oil
- 1 teaspoon garlic powder
- 1 teaspoon paprika
- 1 teaspoon dried basil
- A pinch of lemon-pepper seasoning
- Garlic Aioli:
- 2 garlic cloves, minced
- 1 tablespoon mayonnaise
- Juice of ½ lemon
- 1 teaspoon extra-virgin olive oil
- Salt and pepper, to taste

Directions:
1. On a clean work surface, brush both sides of each fillet with the olive oil. Sprinkle with the garlic powder, paprika, basil, and lemon-pepper seasoning. Place the fillets in the baking pan.
2. Slide the baking pan into Rack Position 1, select Convection Bake, set temperature to 400ºF (205ºC), and set time to 15 minutes.
3. Flip the fillets halfway through.
4. Meanwhile, make the garlic aioli: Whisk together the garlic, mayo, lemon juice, olive oil, salt, and pepper in a small bowl until smooth.
5. When cooking is complete, the fish should flake apart with a fork and no longer translucent in the center. Remove the fish from the oven and serve with the garlic aioli on the side.

390.Glazed Tuna And Fruit Kebabs

Servings: 4
Cooking Time: 10 Minutes
Ingredients:
- Kebabs:
- 1 pound (454 g) tuna steaks, cut into 1-inch cubes
- ½ cup canned pineapple chunks, drained, juice reserved
- ½ cup large red grapes
- Marinade:
- 1 tablespoon honey
- 1 teaspoon olive oil
- 2 teaspoons grated fresh ginger
- Pinch cayenne pepper
- Special Equipment:
- 4 metal skewers

Directions:
1. Make the kebabs: Thread, alternating tuna cubes, pineapple chunks, and red grapes, onto the metal skewers.
2. Make the marinade: Whisk together the honey, olive oil, ginger, and cayenne pepper in a small bowl. Brush generously the marinade over the kebabs and allow to sit for 10 minutes.
3. When ready, transfer the kebabs to the air fryer basket.
4. Put the air fryer basket on the baking pan and slide into Rack Position 2, select Air Fry, set temperature to 370ºF (188ºC), and set time to 10 minutes.
5. After 5 minutes, remove from the oven and flip the kebabs and brush with the remaining marinade. Return the pan to the oven and continue cooking for an additional 5 minutes.
6. When cooking is complete, the kebabs should reach an internal temperature of 145ºF (63ºC) on a meat thermometer. Remove from the oven and discard any remaining marinade. Serve hot.

391.Lobster Grandma's Easy To Cook Wontons

Ingredients:
- 1 ½ cup all-purpose flour
- ½ tsp. salt
- 5 tbsp. water
- For filling:
- 2 cups minced lobster
- 2 tbsp. oil
- 2 tsp. ginger-garlic paste
- 2 tsp. soya sauce
- 2 tsp. vinegar

Directions:

1. Squeeze the dough and cover it with plastic wrap and set aside. Next, cook the ingredients for the filling and try to ensure that the lobster is covered well with the sauce.
2. Roll the dough and place the filling in the center. Now, wrap the dough to cover the filling and pinch the edges together.
3. Pre heat the oven at 200° F for 5 minutes. Place the wontons in the fry basket and close it. Let them cook at the same temperature for another 20 minutes. Recommended sides are chili sauce or ketchup.

392.Baked Tilapia

Servings: 4
Cooking Time: 10 Minutes
Ingredients:
- 1 1/4 lbs tilapia fillets
- 2 tsp onion powder
- 2 tbsp olive oil
- 1/2 tsp garlic powder
- 1/2 tsp dried thyme
- 1/2 tsp oregano
- 1/2 tsp chili powder
- 2 tbsp sweet paprika
- 1 tsp pepper
- 1/2 tsp salt

Directions:
1. Fit the oven with the rack in position
2. Brush fish fillets with oil and place in baking dish.
3. Mix together spices and sprinkle over the fish fillets.
4. Set to bake at 425 F for 15 minutes. After 5 minutes place the baking dish in the preheated oven.
5. Serve and enjoy.
Nutrition Info: Calories 195 Fat 8.9 g Carbohydrates 3.9 g Sugar 0.9 g Protein 27.2 g Cholesterol 69 mg

393.Carp Best Homemade Croquette

Ingredients:
- 1 lb. Carp filets
- 3 onions chopped
- 5 green chilies-roughly chopped
- 1 ½ tbsp. ginger paste
- 1 ½ tsp garlic paste
- 1 ½ tsp salt
- 3 tsp lemon juice
- 2 tsp garam masala
- 4 tbsp. chopped coriander
- 3 tbsp. cream
- 2 tbsp. coriander powder
- 4 tbsp. fresh mint chopped

- 3 tbsp. chopped capsicum
- 3 eggs
- 2 ½ tbsp. white sesame seeds

Directions:
1. Take all the ingredients mentioned under the first heading and mix them in a bowl. Grind them thoroughly to make a smooth paste. Take the eggs in a different bowl and beat them. Add a pinch of salt and leave them aside. Mold the fish mixture into small balls and flatten them into round and flat Best Homemade Croquettes. Dip these Best Homemade Croquettes in the egg and salt mixture and then in the mixture of breadcrumbs and sesame seeds.
2. Leave these Best Homemade Croquettes in the fridge for an hour or so to set. Pre heat the oven at 160 degrees Fahrenheit for around 5 minutes. Place the Best Homemade Croquettes in the basket and let them cook for another 25 minutes at the same temperature. Turn the Best Homemade Croquettes over in between the cooking process to get a uniform cook. Serve the Best Homemade Croquettes with mint sauce.

394.Spinach Scallops

Servings: 2
Cooking Time: 10 Minutes
Ingredients:
- 8 sea scallops
- 1 tbsp fresh basil, chopped
- 1 tbsp tomato paste
- 3/4 cup heavy cream
- 12 oz frozen spinach, thawed and drained
- 1 tsp garlic, minced
- 1/2 tsp pepper
- 1/2 tsp salt

Directions:
1. Fit the oven with the rack in position
2. Layer spinach in the baking dish.
3. Spray scallops with cooking spray and season with pepper and salt.
4. Place scallops on top of spinach.
5. In a small bowl, mix garlic, basil, tomato paste, whipping cream, pepper, and salt and pour over scallops and spinach.
6. Set to bake at 350 F for 15 minutes. After 5 minutes place the baking dish in the preheated oven.
7. Serve and enjoy.
Nutrition Info: Calories 310 Fat 18.3 g Carbohydrates 12.6 g Sugar 1.7 g Protein 26.5 g Cholesterol 101 mg

395.Basil Tomato Salmon

Servings: 2

Cooking Time: 20 Minutes
Ingredients:
- 2 salmon fillets
- 1 tomato, sliced
- 1 tbsp dried basil
- 2 tbsp parmesan cheese, grated
- 1 tbsp olive oil

Directions:
1. Fit the oven with the rack in position
2. Place salmon fillets in a baking dish.
3. Sprinkle basil on top of salmon fillets.
4. Arrange tomato slices on top of salmon fillets. Drizzle with oil and top with cheese.
5. Set to bake at 375 F for 25 minutes. After 5 minutes place the baking dish in the preheated oven.
6. Serve and enjoy.

Nutrition Info: Calories 324 Fat 19.6 g Carbohydrates 1.5 g Sugar 0.8 g Protein 37.1 g Cholesterol 83 mg

396.Crispy Paprika Fish Fillets(1)

Servings: 4
Cooking Time: 15 Minutes
Ingredients:
- 1/2 cup seasoned breadcrumbs
- 1 tablespoon balsamic vinegar
- 1/2 teaspoon seasoned salt
- 1 teaspoon paprika
- 1/2 teaspoon ground black pepper
- 1 teaspoon celery seed
- 2 fish fillets, halved
- 1 egg, beaten

Directions:
1. Preparing the Ingredients. Add the breadcrumbs, vinegar, salt, paprika, ground black pepper, and celery seeds to your food processor. Process for about 30 seconds.
2. Coat the fish fillets with the beaten egg; then, coat them with the breadcrumbs mixture.
3. Air Frying. Cook at 350 degrees F for about 15 minutes.

397.Greek Cod With Asparagus

Servings: 2
Cooking Time: 20 Minutes
Ingredients:
- 1 lb cod, cut into 4 pieces
- 8 asparagus spears
- 1 leek, sliced
- 1 onion, quartered
- 2 tomatoes, halved
- 1/2 tsp oregano
- 1/2 tsp red chili flakes
- 1/2 cup olives, chopped
- 2 tbsp olive oil
- 1/4 tsp pepper
- 1/4 tsp salt

Directions:
1. Fit the oven with the rack in position
2. Arrange fish pieces, olives, asparagus, leek, onion, and tomatoes in a baking dish.
3. Season with oregano, chili flakes, pepper, and salt and drizzle with olive oil.
4. Set to bake at 400 F for 25 minutes. After 5 minutes place the baking dish in the preheated oven.
5. Serve and enjoy.

Nutrition Info: Calories 489 Fat 20.2 g Carbohydrates 22.5 g Sugar 9.1 g Protein 56.6 g Cholesterol 125 mg

398.Chili Prawns

Servings: 2
Cooking Time: 8 Minutes
Ingredients:
- 8 prawns, cleaned
- Salt and black pepper, to taste
- ½ teaspoon ground cayenne pepper
- ½ teaspoon garlic powder
- ½ teaspoon ground cumin
- ½ teaspoon red chili flakes
- Cooking spray

Directions:
1. Spritz the air fryer basket with cooking spray.
2. Toss the remaining ingredients in a large bowl until the prawns are well coated.
3. Spread the coated prawns evenly in the basket and spray them with cooking spray.
4. Put the air fryer basket on the baking pan and slide into Rack Position 2, select Air Fry, set temperature to 340ºF (171ºC), and set time to 8 minutes.
5. Flip the prawns halfway through the cooking time.
6. When cooking is complete, the prawns should be pink. Remove the prawns from the oven to a plate.

399.Cajun Catfish Cakes With Cheese

Servings: 4
Cooking Time: 15 Minutes
Ingredients:
- 2 catfish fillets
- 3 ounces (85 g) butter
- 1 cup shredded Parmesan cheese
- 1 cup shredded Swiss cheese
- ½ cup buttermilk
- 1 teaspoon baking powder

- 1 teaspoon baking soda
- 1 teaspoon Cajun seasoning

Directions:

1. Bring a pot of salted water to a boil. Add the catfish fillets to the boiling water and let them boil for 5 minutes until they become opaque.
2. Remove the fillets from the pot to a mixing bowl and flake them into small pieces with a fork.
3. Add the remaining ingredients to the bowl of fish and stir until well incorporated.
4. Divide the fish mixture into 12 equal portions and shape each portion into a patty. Place the patties in the air fryer basket.
5. Put the air fryer basket on the baking pan and slide into Rack Position 2, select Air Fry, set temperature to 380ºF (193ºC), and set time to 15 minutes.
6. Flip the patties halfway through the cooking time.
7. When cooking is complete, the patties should be golden brown and cooked through. Remove from the oven. Let the patties sit for 5 minutes and serve.

MEATLESS RECIPES

400.Yam French Cuisine Galette

Ingredients:
- 1 ½ tbsp. lemon juice
- Salt and pepper to taste
- 2 cups minced yam
- 3 tsp. ginger finely chopped
- 1-2 tbsp. fresh coriander leaves
- 2 or 3 green chilies finely chopped

Directions:
1. Mix the ingredients in a clean bowl.
2. Mold this mixture into round and flat French Cuisine Galettes.
3. Wet the French Cuisine Galettes slightly with water.
4. Pre heat the oven at 160 degrees Fahrenheit for 5 minutes. Place the French Cuisine Galettes in the fry basket and let them cook for another 25 minutes at the same temperature. Keep rolling them over to get a uniform cook. Serve either with mint sauce or ketchup.

401.Classic Baked Potatoes

Servings: 4
Cooking Time: 30 Minutes
Ingredients:
- 1 lb potatoes
- 2 garlic cloves, minced
- Salt and black pepper to taste
- 1 tsp rosemary
- 1 tsp butter, melted

Directions:
1. Preheat Breville oven to 360 F on AirFry function. Prick the potatoes with a fork. Place into frying basket and press Start. Cook for 25 minutes. Cut the potatoes in half and top with butter and rosemary. Season with salt and pepper and serve.

402.Roasted Brussels Sprouts With Parmesan

Servings: 4
Cooking Time: 20 Minutes
Ingredients:
- 1 pound (454 g) fresh Brussels sprouts, trimmed
- 1 tablespoon olive oil
- ½ teaspoon salt
- ⅛ teaspoon pepper
- ¼ cup grated Parmesan cheese

Directions:
1. In a large bowl, combine the Brussels sprouts with olive oil, salt, and pepper and toss until evenly coated.
2. Spread the Brussels sprouts evenly in the air fryer basket.
3. Put the air fryer basket on the baking pan and slide into Rack Position 2, select Air Fry, set temperature to 330ºF (166ºC), and set time to 20 minutes.
4. Stir the Brussels sprouts twice during cooking.
5. When cooking is complete, the Brussels sprouts should be golden brown and crisp. Sprinkle the grated Parmesan cheese on top and serve warm.

403.Vegetable And Cheese Stuffed Tomatoes

Servings: 4
Cooking Time: 18 Minutes
Ingredients:
- 4 medium beefsteak tomatoes, rinsed
- ½ cup grated carrot
- 1 medium onion, chopped
- 1 garlic clove, minced
- 2 teaspoons olive oil
- 2 cups fresh baby spinach
- ¼ cup crumbled low-sodium feta cheese
- ½ teaspoon dried basil

Directions:
1. On your cutting board, cut a thin slice off the top of each tomato. Scoop out a ¼- to ½-inch-thick tomato pulp and place the tomatoes upside down on paper towels to drain. Set aside.
2. Stir together the carrot, onion, garlic, and olive oil in the baking pan.
3. Slide the baking pan into Rack Position 1, select Convection Bake, set temperature to 350ºF (180ºC) and set time to 5 minutes.
4. Stir the vegetables halfway through.
5. When cooking is complete, the carrot should be crisp-tender.
6. Remove from the oven and stir in the spinach, feta cheese, and basil.
7. Spoon ¼ of the vegetable mixture into each tomato and transfer the stuffed tomatoes to the oven. Set time to 13 minutes.
8. When cooking is complete, the filling should be hot and the tomatoes should be lightly caramelized.
9. Let the tomatoes cool for 5 minutes and serve.

404.Cheese & Vegetable Pizza

Servings: 1
Cooking Time: 15 Minutes
Ingredients:
- 1 tbsp tomato paste
- ¼ cup mozzarella cheese, grated

- 1 tbsp sweet corn, cooked
- 4 zucchini slices
- 4 eggplant slices
- 4 red onion rings
- ½ green bell pepper, chopped
- 3 cherry tomatoes, quartered
- 1 tortilla
- ¼ tsp oregano

Directions:
1. Preheat Breville on Pizza function to 350 F. Spread the tomato paste on the tortilla. Top with zucchini and eggplant slices first, then green peppers, and onion rings.
2. Arrange the cherry tomatoes on top and scatter the corn. Sprinkle with oregano and top with mozzarella cheeses. Press Start and cook for 10-12 minutes. Serve warm.

405.Vegetable Au Gratin

Servings: 3
Cooking Time: 30 Minutes
Ingredients:
- 1 cup cubed eggplant
- ¼ cup chopped red pepper
- ¼ cup chopped green pepper
- ¼ cup chopped onion
- ⅓ cup chopped tomatoes
- 1 clove garlic, minced
- 1 tbsp sliced pimiento-stuffed olives
- 1 tsp capers
- ¼ tsp dried basil
- ¼ tsp dried marjoram
- Salt and black pepper to taste
- ¼ cup grated mozzarella cheese
- 1 tbsp breadcrumbs

Directions:
1. In a bowl, add eggplant, peppers, onion, tomatoes, olives, garlic, basil, marjoram, capers, salt, and black pepper. Lightly grease a baking tray with cooking spray. Add in the vegetable mixture and spread it evenly. Sprinkle mozzarella cheese on top and cover with breadcrumbs. Cook in your for 20 minutes on Bake function at 360 F. Serve.

406.Homemade Cheese Ravioli

Servings: 4
Cooking Time: 15 Minutes
Ingredients:
- 1 package cheese ravioli
- 2 cup Italian breadcrumbs
- ¼ cup Parmesan cheese, grated
- 1 cup buttermilk
- 1 tsp olive oil

- ¼ tsp garlic powder

Directions:
1. Preheat on Air Fry function to 390 F. In a small bowl, combine breadcrumbs, Parmesan cheese, garlic powder, and olive oil. Dip the ravioli in the buttermilk and then coat them with the breadcrumb mixture.
2. Line the Air Fryer pan with parchment paper and arrange the ravioli on it. Cook for 5 minutes. Serve the ravioli with marinara sauce.

407.Honey-glazed Roasted Veggies

Servings: 3 Cups
Cooking Time: 20 Minutes
Ingredients:
- Glaze:
- 2 tablespoons raw honey
- 2 teaspoons minced garlic
- ¼ teaspoon dried marjoram
- ¼ teaspoon dried basil
- ¼ teaspoon dried oregano
- ⅛ teaspoon dried sage
- ⅛ teaspoon dried rosemary
- ⅛ teaspoon dried thyme
- ½ teaspoon salt
- ¼ teaspoon ground black pepper
- Veggies:
- 3 to 4 medium red potatoes, cut into 1- to 2-inch pieces
- 1 small zucchini, cut into 1- to 2-inch pieces
- 1 small carrot, sliced into ¼-inch rounds
- 1 (10.5-ounce / 298-g) package cherry tomatoes, halved
- 1 cup sliced mushrooms
- 3 tablespoons olive oil

Directions:
1. Combine the honey, garlic, marjoram, basil, oregano, sage, rosemary, thyme, salt, and pepper in a small bowl and stir to mix well. Set aside.
2. Place the red potatoes, zucchini, carrot, cherry tomatoes, and mushroom in a large bowl. Drizzle with the olive oil and toss to coat.
3. Pour the veggies into the baking pan.
4. Slide the baking pan into Rack Position 2, select Roast, set temperature to 380ºF (193ºC) and set time to 15 minutes.
5. Stir the veggies halfway through.
6. When cooking is complete, the vegetables should be tender.
7. When ready, transfer the roasted veggies to the large bowl. Pour the honey mixture over the veggies, tossing to coat.
8. Spread out the veggies in the baking pan.
9. Increase the temperature to 390ºF (199ºC) and set time to 5 minutes on Roast.

10. When cooking is complete, the veggies should be tender and glazed. Serve warm.

408.Air Fried Winter Vegetables

Servings: 2
Cooking Time: 16 Minutes
Ingredients:
- 1 parsnip, sliced
- 1 cup sliced butternut squash
- 1 small red onion, cut into wedges
- ½ chopped celery stalk
- 1 tablespoon chopped fresh thyme
- 2 teaspoons olive oil
- Salt and black pepper, to taste

Directions:
1. Toss all the ingredients in a large bowl until the vegetables are well coated.
2. Transfer the vegetables to the air fryer basket.
3. Put the air fryer basket on the baking pan and slide into Rack Position 2, select Air Fry, set temperature to 380ºF (193ºC), and set time to 16 minutes.
4. Stir the vegetables halfway through the cooking time.
5. When cooking is complete, the vegetables should be golden brown and tender. Remove from the oven and serve warm.

409.Roasted Butternut Squash With Maple Syrup

Servings: 4
Cooking Time: 30 Minutes
Ingredients:
- 1 lb butternut squash
- 1 tsp dried rosemary
- 2 tbsp maple syrup
- Salt to taste

Directions:
1. Place the squash on a cutting board and peel. Cut in half and remove the seeds and pulp. Slice into wedges and season with salt. Spray with cooking spray and sprinkle with rosemary.
2. Preheat Breville on AirFry function to 350 F. Transfer the wedges to the greased basket without overlapping. Press Start and cook for 20 minutes. Serve drizzled with maple syrup.

410.Masala French Fries

Ingredients:
- 2 medium sized potatoes peeled and cut into thick pieces lengthwise
- 1 tbsp. olive oil
- 1 tsp. mixed herbs
- 1 tbsp. lemon juice
- ½ tsp. red chili flakes
- A pinch of salt to taste

Directions:
1. Boil the potatoes and blanch them. Cut the potato into Oregano Fingers. Mix the ingredients for the marinade and add the potato Oregano Fingers to it making sure that they are coated well.
2. Pre heat the oven for around 5 minutes at 300 Fahrenheit. Take out the basket of the fryer and place the potato Oregano Fingers in them. Close the basket.
3. Now keep the fryer at 200 Fahrenheit for 20 or 25 minutes. In between the process, toss the fries twice or thrice so that they get cooked properly.

411.Stuffed Peppers With Beans And Rice

Servings: 4
Cooking Time: 18 Minutes
Ingredients:
- 4 medium red, green, or yellow bell peppers, halved and deseeded
- 4 tablespoons extra-virgin olive oil, divided
- ½ teaspoon kosher salt, divided
- 1 (15-ounce / 425-g) can chickpeas
- 1½ cups cooked white rice
- ½ cup diced roasted red peppers
- ¼ cup chopped parsley
- ½ small onion, finely chopped
- 3 garlic cloves, minced
- ½ teaspoon cumin
- ¼ teaspoon freshly ground black pepper
- ¾ cup panko bread crumbs

Directions:
1. Brush the peppers inside and out with 1 tablespoon of olive oil. Season the insides with ¼ teaspoon of kosher salt. Arrange the peppers in the air fryer basket, cut side up.
2. Place the chickpeas with their liquid into a large bowl. Lightly mash the beans with a potato masher. Sprinkle with the remaining ¼ teaspoon of kosher salt and 1 tablespoon of olive oil. Add the rice, red peppers, parsley, onion, garlic, cumin, and black pepper to the bowl and stir to incorporate.
3. Divide the mixture among the bell pepper halves.
4. Stir together the remaining 2 tablespoons of olive oil and panko in a small bowl. Top the pepper halves with the panko mixture.
5. Put the air fryer basket on the baking pan and slide into Rack Position 2, select Roast, set temperature to 375ºF (190ºC), and set time to 18 minutes.
6. When done, the peppers should be slightly wrinkled, and the panko should be golden brown.
7. Remove from the oven and serve on a plate.

412.Black Gram French Cuisine Galette

Ingredients:
- 2 or 3 green chilies finely chopped
- 1 ½ tbsp. lemon juice
- Salt and pepper to taste
- 2 cup black gram
- 2 medium potatoes boiled and mashed
- 1 ½ cup coarsely crushed peanuts
- 3 tsp. ginger finely chopped
- 1-2 tbsp. fresh coriander leaves

Directions:
1. Mix the ingredients in a clean bowl.
2. Mold this mixture into round and flat French Cuisine Galettes.
3. Wet the French Cuisine Galettes slightly with water.
4. Pre heat the oven at 160 degrees Fahrenheit for 5 minutes. Place the French Cuisine Galettes in the fry basket and let them cook for another 25 minutes at the same temperature. Keep rolling them over to get a uniform cook. Serve either with mint sauce or ketchup.

413.Cumin Sweet Potatoes Wedges

Servings: 4
Cooking Time: 30 Minutes
Ingredients:
- ½ tsp garlic powder
- ½ tsp cayenne pepper powder
- ¼ tsp ground cumin
- 3 tbsp olive oil
- 3 sweet potatoes, cut into ½-inch thick wedges
- 2 tbsp fresh parsley, chopped
- Sea salt to taste

Directions:
1. In a bowl, mix salt, garlic powder, cayenne pepper powder, and cumin. Whisk in olive oil and coat in the potatoes. Arrange them on the basket, without overcrowding and press Start. Cook for 20-25 minutes at 380 F on AirFry function. Sprinkle with parsley and sea salt and serve.

414.Mushroom Pasta

Ingredients:
- 2 cups sliced mushroom
- 2 tbsp. all-purpose flour
- 2 cups of milk
- 1 tsp. dried oregano
- ½ tsp. dried basil
- ½ tsp. dried parsley

- 1 cup pasta
- 1 ½ tbsp. olive oil
- A pinch of salt
- For tossing pasta:
- 1 ½ tbsp. olive oil
- Salt and pepper to taste
- ½ tsp. oregano
- ½ tsp. basil
- 2 tbsp. olive oil
- Salt and pepper to taste

Directions:
1. Boil the pasta and sieve it when done. You will need to toss the pasta in the ingredients mentioned above and set aside.
2. For the sauce, add the ingredients to a pan and bring the ingredients to a boil. Stir the sauce and continue to simmer to make a thicker sauce. Add the pasta to the sauce and transfer this into a glass bowl garnished with cheese.
3. Pre heat the oven at 160 degrees for 5 minutes. Place the bowl in the basket and close it. Let it continue to cook at the same temperature for 10 minutes more. Keep stirring the pasta in between.

415.Asparagus French Cuisine Galette

Ingredients:
- 1 ½ tbsp. lemon juice
- Salt and pepper to taste
- 2 cups minced asparagus
- 3 tsp. ginger finely chopped
- 1-2 tbsp. fresh coriander leaves
- 2 or 3 green chilies finely chopped

Directions:
1. Mix the ingredients in a clean bowl.
2. Mold this mixture into round and flat French Cuisine Galettes.
3. Wet the French Cuisine Galettes slightly with water.
4. Pre heat the oven at 160 degrees Fahrenheit for 5 minutes. Place the French Cuisine Galettes in the fry basket and let them cook for another 25 minutes at the same temperature. Keep rolling them over to get a uniform cook. Serve either with mint sauce or ketchup.

416.Cottage Cheese Homemade Fried Sticks

Ingredients:
- One or two poppadums'
- 4 or 5 tbsp. corn flour
- 1 cup of water
- 2 cups cottage cheese
- 1 big lemon-juiced

- 1 tbsp. ginger-garlic paste
- For seasoning, use salt and red chili powder in small amounts
- ½ tsp. carom

Directions:

1. Take the cottage cheese. Cut it into long pieces. Now, make a mixture of lemon juice, red chili powder, salt, ginger garlic paste and carom to use as a marinade. Let the cottage cheese pieces marinate in the mixture for some time and then roll them in dry corn flour. Leave them aside for around 20 minutes.

2. Take the poppadum into a pan and roast them. Once they are cooked, crush them into very small pieces. Now take another container and pour around 100 ml of water into it. Dissolve 2 tbsp. of corn flour in this water. Dip the cottage cheese pieces in this solution of corn flour and roll them on to the pieces of crushed poppadum so that the poppadum sticks to the cottage cheese

3. . Pre heat the oven for 10 minutes at 290 Fahrenheit. Then open the basket of the fryer and place the cottage cheese pieces inside it. Close the basket properly. Let the fryer stay at 160 degrees for another 20 minutes. Halfway through, open the basket and toss the cottage cheese around a bit to allow for uniform cooking. Once they are done, you can serve it either with ketchup or mint sauce. Another recommended side is mint sauce.

417.Chickpea Fritters

Servings: 4
Cooking Time: 10 Minutes
Ingredients:

- Nonstick cooking spray
- 1 cup chickpeas, cooked
- 1 onion, chopped
- ¼ tsp salt
- ¼ tsp pepper
- ¼ tsp turmeric
- ¼ tsp coriander

Directions:

1. Place the baking pan in position 2. Lightly spray the fryer basket with cooking spray.

2. Add the onion to a food processor and pulse until finely diced.

3. Add remaining ingredients and pulse until combined but not pureed.

4. Form the mixture into 8 patties and place them in the fryer basket, these may need to be cooked in two batches.

5. Place the basket in the oven and set to air fry on 350°F for 10 minutes. Cook fritters until golden brown and crispy, turning over halfway through cooking time. Serve with your favorite dipping sauce.

Nutrition Info: Calories 101, Total Fat 1g, Saturated Fat 0g, Total Carbs 14g, Net Carbs 10g, Protein 4g, Sugar 3g, Fiber 4g, Sodium 149mg, Potassium 159mg, Phosphorus 77mg

418.Dal Mint Spicy Lemon Kebab

Ingredients:

- 2 tsp. coriander powder
- 1 ½ tbsp. chopped coriander
- ½ tsp. dried mango powder
- 1 cup dry breadcrumbs
- ¼ tsp. black salt
- 1-2 tbsp. all-purpose flour for coating purposes
- 1-2 tbsp. mint (finely chopped)
- 1 cup chickpeas
- Half inch ginger grated or one and a half tsp. of ginger-garlic paste
- 1-2 green chilies chopped finely
- ¼ tsp. red chili powder
- A pinch of salt to taste
- ½ tsp. roasted cumin powder
- 1 onion that has been finely chopped
- ½ cup milk

Directions:

1. Take an open vessel. Boil the chickpeas in the vessel until their texture becomes soft. Make sure that they do not become soggy. Now take this chickpea into another container. Add the grated ginger and the cut green chilies.

2. Grind this mixture until it becomes a thick paste. Keep adding water as and when required. Now add the onions, mint, the breadcrumbs and all the various masalas required. Mix this well until you get a soft dough. Now take small balls of this mixture (about the size of a lemon) and mold them into the shape of flat and round kebabs.

3. Here is where the milk comes into play. Pour a very small amount of milk onto each kebab to wet it. Now roll the kebab in the dry breadcrumbs. Pre heat the oven for 5 minutes at 300 Fahrenheit. Take out the basket.

4. Arrange the kebabs in the basket leaving gaps between them so that no two kebabs are touching each other. Keep the fryer at 340 Fahrenheit for around half an hour. Half way through the cooking process, turn the kebabs over so that they can be cooked properly. Recommended sides for this dish are mint sauce, tomato ketchup or yoghurt sauce.

419.Veggie Mix Fried Chips

Servings: 4
Cooking Time: 45 Minutes
Ingredients:

- 1 large eggplant, cut into strips
- 5 potatoes, peeled and cut into strips
- 3 zucchinis, cut into strips
- ½ cup cornstarch
- ½ cup olive oil
- Salt to taste

Directions:

1. Preheat Breville on AirFry function to 390 F. In a bowl, stir cornstarch, ½ cup of water, salt, pepper, olive oil, eggplants, zucchini, and potatoes. Place the veggie mixture in the basket and press Start. Cook for 12 minutes. Serve warm.

420.Tortellini With Veggies And Parmesan

Servings: 4
Cooking Time: 16 Minutes
Ingredients:

- 8 ounces (227 g) sugar snap peas, trimmed
- ½ pound (227 g) asparagus, trimmed and cut into 1-inch pieces
- 2 teaspoons kosher salt or 1 teaspoon fine salt, divided
- 1 tablespoon extra-virgin olive oil
- 1½ cups water
- 1 (20-ounce / 340-g) package frozen cheese tortellini
- 2 garlic cloves, minced
- 1 cup heavy (whipping) cream
- 1 cup cherry tomatoes, halved
- ½ cup grated Parmesan cheese
- ¼ cup chopped fresh parsley or basil
- Add the peas and asparagus to a large bowl. Add ½ teaspoon of kosher salt and the olive oil and toss until well coated. Place the veggies in the baking pan.

Directions:

1. Slide the baking pan into Rack Position 1, select Convection Bake, set the temperature to 450ºF (235ºC), and set the time for 4 minutes.
2. Meanwhile, dissolve 1 teaspoon of kosher salt in the water.
3. Once cooking is complete, remove the pan from the oven and place the tortellini in the pan. Pour the salted water over the tortellini. Put the pan back to the oven.
4. Slide the baking pan into Rack Position 1, select Convection Bake, set temperature to 450ºF (235ºC), and set time for 7 minutes.
5. Meantime, stir together the garlic, heavy cream, and remaining ½ teaspoon of kosher salt in a small bowl.
6. Once cooking is complete, remove the pan from the oven. Blot off any remaining water with a paper towel. Gently stir the ingredients. Drizzle the cream over and top with the tomatoes.

7. Slide the baking pan into Rack Position 2, select Roast, set the temperature to 375ºF (190ºC), and set the time for 5 minutes.
8. After 4 minutes, remove from the oven.
9. Add the Parmesan cheese and stir until the cheese is melted
10. Serve topped with the parsley.

421.Mozzarella Eggplant Patties

Servings: 1
Cooking Time: 10 Minutes
Ingredients:

- 1 hamburger bun
- 1 eggplant, sliced
- 1 mozzarella slice, chopped
- 1 red onion cut into 3 rings
- 1 lettuce leaf
- ½ tbsp tomato sauce
- 1 pickle, sliced

Directions:

1. Preheat on Bake function to 330 F. Place the eggplant slices in a greased baking tray and cook for 6 minutes. Take out the tray and top the eggplant with mozzarella cheese and cook for 30 more seconds. Spread tomato sauce on one half of the bun. Place the lettuce leaf on top of the sauce. Place the cheesy eggplant on top of the lettuce. Top with onion rings and pickles and then with the other bun half to serve.

422.Cottage Cheese Pops

Ingredients:

- 1 tsp. dry basil
- ½ cup hung curd
- 1 tsp. lemon juice
- 1 cup cottage cheese cut into 2" cubes
- 1 ½ tsp. garlic paste
- Salt and pepper to taste
- 1 tsp. dry oregano
- 1 tsp. red chili flakes

Directions:

1. Cut the cottage cheese into thick and long rectangular pieces.
2. Add the rest of the ingredients into a separate bowl and mix them well to get a consistent mixture.
3. Dip the cottage cheese pieces in the above mixture and leave them aside for some time.
4. Pre heat the oven at 180° C for around 5 minutes. Place the coated cottage cheese pieces in the fry basket and close it properly. Let them cook at the same temperature for 20 more minutes. Keep turning them over in the basket so that they are cooked properly. Serve with tomato ketchup.

423.Speedy Vegetable Pizza

Servings: 1
Cooking Time: 15 Minutes
Ingredients:
- 1 ½ tbsp tomato paste
- ¼ cup grated cheddar cheese
- ¼ cup grated mozzarella cheese
- 1 tbsp cooked sweet corn
- 4 zucchini slices
- 4 eggplant slices
- 4 red onion rings
- ½ green bell pepper, chopped
- 3 cherry tomatoes, quartered
- 1 pizza crust
- ¼ tsp basil
- ¼ tsp oregano

Directions:
1. Preheat on Bake function to 350 F. Spread the tomato paste on the pizza crust. Top with zucchini and eggplant slices first, then green peppers, and onion rings. Cover with cherry tomatoes and scatter the corn. Sprinkle with oregano and basil and sprinkle with cheddar and mozzarella cheeses. Cook for 10-12 minutes until golden brown on top. Serve.

424.Herbed Broccoli With Cheese

Servings: 4
Cooking Time: 18 Minutes
Ingredients:
- 1 large-sized head broccoli, stemmed and cut into small florets
- 2½ tablespoons canola oil
- 2 teaspoons dried basil
- 2 teaspoons dried rosemary
- Salt and ground black pepper, to taste
- $^1/_3$ cup grated yellow cheese

Directions:
1. Bring a pot of lightly salted water to a boil. Add the broccoli florets to the boiling water and let boil for about 3 minutes.
2. Drain the broccoli florets well and transfer to a large bowl. Add the canola oil, basil, rosemary, salt, and black pepper to the bowl and toss until the broccoli is fully coated. Place the broccoli in the air fryer basket.
3. Put the air fryer basket on the baking pan and slide into Rack Position 2, select Air Fry, set temperature to 390ºF (199ºC), and set time to 15 minutes.
4. Stir the broccoli halfway through the cooking time.

5. When cooking is complete, the broccoli should be crisp. Serve the broccoli warm with grated cheese sprinkled on top.

425.Teriyaki Cauliflower

Servings: 4
Cooking Time: 14 Minutes
Ingredients:
- ½ cup soy sauce
- $^1/_3$ cup water
- 1 tablespoon brown sugar
- 1 teaspoon sesame oil
- 1 teaspoon cornstarch
- 2 cloves garlic, chopped
- ½ teaspoon chili powder
- 1 big cauliflower head, cut into florets

Directions:
1. Make the teriyaki sauce: In a small bowl, whisk together the soy sauce, water, brown sugar, sesame oil, cornstarch, garlic, and chili powder until well combined.
2. Place the cauliflower florets in a large bowl and drizzle the top with the prepared teriyaki sauce and toss to coat well.
3. Put the cauliflower florets in the air fryer basket.
4. Put the air fryer basket on the baking pan and slide into Rack Position 2, select Air Fry, set temperature to 340ºF (171ºC) and set time to 14 minutes.
5. Stir the cauliflower halfway through.
6. When cooking is complete, the cauliflower should be crisp-tender.
7. Let the cauliflower cool for 5 minutes before serving.

426.Grandma´s Ratatouille

Servings: 2
Cooking Time: 30 Minutes
Ingredients:
- 1 tbsp olive oil
- 3 Roma tomatoes, thinly sliced
- 2 garlic cloves, minced
- 1 zucchini, thinly sliced
- 2 yellow bell peppers, sliced
- 1 tbsp vinegar
- 2 tbsp herbs de Provence
- Salt and black pepper to taste

Directions:
1. Preheat Breville on AirFry function to 390 F. Place all ingredients in a bowl. Season with salt and pepper and stir to coat. Arrange the vegetable on a baking dish and place in the Breville oven. Cook for

15 minutes, shaking occasionally. Let sit for 5 more minutes after the timer goes off.

427. Cashew Cauliflower With Yogurt Sauce

Servings: 2
Cooking Time: 12 Minutes
Ingredients:
- 4 cups cauliflower florets (about half a large head)
- 1 tablespoon olive oil
- 1 teaspoon curry powder
- Salt, to taste
- ½ cup toasted, chopped cashews, for garnish
- Yogurt Sauce:
- ¼ cup plain yogurt
- 2 tablespoons sour cream
- 1 teaspoon honey
- 1 teaspoon lemon juice
- Pinch cayenne pepper
- Salt, to taste
- 1 tablespoon chopped fresh cilantro, plus leaves for garnish

Directions:
1. In a large mixing bowl, toss the cauliflower florets with the olive oil, curry powder, and salt.
2. Place the cauliflower florets in the air fryer basket.
3. Put the air fryer basket on the baking pan and slide into Rack Position 2, select Air Fry, set temperature to 400ºF (205ºC) and set time to 12 minutes.
4. Stir the cauliflower florets twice during cooking.
5. When cooking is complete, the cauliflower should be golden brown.
6. Meanwhile, mix all the ingredients for the yogurt sauce in a small bowl and whisk to combine.
7. Remove the cauliflower from the oven and drizzle with the yogurt sauce. Scatter the toasted cashews and cilantro on top and serve immediately.

428. Apricot Spicy Lemon Kebab

Ingredients:
- 3 tsp. lemon juice
- 2 tsp. garam masala
- 3 eggs
- 2 ½ tbsp. white sesame seeds
- 2 cups fresh apricots
- 3 onions chopped
- 5 green chilies-roughly chopped
- 1 ½ tbsp. ginger paste
- 1 ½ tsp. garlic paste
- 1 ½ tsp. salt

Directions:
1. Grind the ingredients except for the egg and form a smooth paste. Coat the apricots in the paste. Now, beat the eggs and add a little salt to it.
2. Dip the coated apricots in the egg mixture and then transfer to the sesame seeds and coat the apricots well. Place the vegetables on a stick.
3. Pre heat the oven at 160 degrees Fahrenheit for around 5 minutes. Place the sticks in the basket and let them cook for another 25 minutes at the same temperature. Turn the sticks over in between the cooking process to get a uniform cook.

429. Garlicky Sesame Carrots

Servings: 4 To 6
Cooking Time: 16 Minutes
Ingredients:
- 1 pound (454 g) baby carrots
- 1 tablespoon sesame oil
- ½ teaspoon dried dill
- Pinch salt
- Freshly ground black pepper, to taste
- 6 cloves garlic, peeled
- 3 tablespoons sesame seeds

Directions:
1. In a medium bowl, drizzle the baby carrots with the sesame oil. Sprinkle with the dill, salt, and pepper and toss to coat well.
2. Place the baby carrots in the air fryer basket.
3. Put the air fryer basket on the baking pan and slide into Rack Position 2, select Roast, set temperature to 380ºF (193ºC), and set time to 16 minutes.
4. After 8 minutes, remove from the oven and stir in the garlic. Return the pan to the oven and continue roasting for 8 minutes more.
5. When cooking is complete, the carrots should be lightly browned. Remove from the oven and serve sprinkled with the sesame seeds.

430. Stuffed Portobellos With Peppers And Cheese

Servings: 4
Cooking Time: 15 Minutes
Ingredients:
- 4 tablespoons sherry vinegar or white wine vinegar
- 6 garlic cloves, minced, divided
- 1 tablespoon fresh thyme leaves
- 1 teaspoon Dijon mustard
- 1 teaspoon kosher salt, divided
- ¼ cup plus 3¼ teaspoons extra-virgin olive oil, divided

- 8 portobello mushroom caps, each about 3 inches across, patted dry
- 1 small red or yellow bell pepper, thinly sliced
- 1 small green bell pepper, thinly sliced
- 1 small onion, thinly sliced
- ¼ teaspoon red pepper flakes
- Freshly ground black pepper, to taste
- 4 ounces (113 g) shredded Fontina cheese

Directions:
1. Stir together the vinegar, 4 minced garlic cloves, thyme, mustard, and ½ teaspoon of kosher salt in a small bowl. Slowly pour in ¼ cup of olive oil, whisking constantly, or until an emulsion is formed. Reserve 2 tablespoons of the marinade and set aside.
2. Put the mushrooms in a resealable plastic bag and pour in the marinade. Seal and shake the bag, coating the mushrooms in the marinade. Transfer the mushrooms to the baking pan, gill-side down.
3. Put the remaining 2 minced garlic cloves, bell peppers, onion, red pepper flakes, remaining ½ teaspoon of salt, and black pepper in a medium bowl. Drizzle with the remaining 3¼ teaspoons of olive oil and toss well. Transfer the bell pepper mixture to the pan.
4. Slide the baking pan into Rack Position 2, select Roast, set temperature to 375ºF (190ºC), and set time to 12 minutes.
5. After 7 minutes, remove the pan and stir the peppers and flip the mushrooms. Return the pan to the oven and continue cooking for 5 minutes.
6. Remove from the oven and place the pepper mixture onto a cutting board and coarsely chop.
7. Brush both sides of the mushrooms with the reserved 2 tablespoons marinade. Stuff the caps evenly with the pepper mixture. Scatter the cheese on top.
8. Select Convection Broil, set temperature to High, and set time to 3 minutes.
9. When done, the mushrooms should be tender and the cheese should be melted.
10. Serve warm.

431.Vegan Beetroot Chips

Servings: 2
Cooking Time: 9 Minutes
Ingredients:
- 4 cups golden beetroot slices
- 2 tbsp olive oil
- 1 tbsp yeast flakes
- 1 tsp vegan seasoning
- Salt to taste

Directions:
1. In a bowl, add the oil, beetroot slices, vegan seasoning, and yeast and mix well. Dump the coated chips in the basket. Set the heat to 370 F and press Start. Cook on AirFry function for14-16 minutes, shaking once halfway through. Serve.

432.Cauliflower Gnocchi's

Ingredients:
- 2 tbsp. oil
- 2 tsp. ginger-garlic paste
- 2 tsp. soya sauce
- 2 tsp. vinegar
- 1 ½ cup all-purpose flour
- ½ tsp. salt
- 5 tbsp. water
- 2 cups grated cauliflower

Directions:
1. Squeeze the dough and cover it with plastic wrap and set aside. Next, cook the ingredients for the filling and try to ensure that the cauliflower is covered well with the sauce.
2. Roll the dough and place the filling in the center. Now, wrap the dough to cover the filling and pinch the edges together.
3. Pre heat the oven at 200° F for 5 minutes. Place the gnocchi's in the fry basket and close it. Let them cook at the same temperature for another 20
4. minutes. Recommended sides are chili sauce or ketchup.

433.Cottage Cheese Gnocchi's

Ingredients:
- 2 tsp. ginger-garlic paste
- 2 tsp. soya sauce
- 2 tsp. vinegar
- 1 ½ cup all-purpose flour
- ½ tsp. salt
- 5 tbsp. water
- 2 cups grated cottage cheese
- 2 tbsp. oil

Directions:
1. Squeeze the dough and cover it with plastic wrap and set aside. Next, cook the ingredients for the filling and try to ensure that the cottage cheese is covered well with the sauce.
2. Roll the dough and place the filling in the center. Now, wrap the dough to cover the filling and pinch the edges together.
3. Pre heat the oven at 200° F for 5 minutes. Place the gnocchi's in the fry basket and close it. Let them cook at the same temperature for another 20 minutes. Recommended sides are chili sauce or ketchup.

434.Yam Spicy Lemon Kebab

Ingredients:
- 2 tsp. garam masala
- 4 tbsp. chopped coriander
- 3 tbsp. cream
- 3 tbsp. chopped capsicum
- 3 eggs
- 2 ½ tbsp. white sesame seeds
- 2 cups sliced yam
- 3 onions chopped
- 5 green chilies-roughly chopped
- 1 ½ tbsp. ginger paste
- 1 ½ tsp. garlic paste
- 1 ½ tsp. salt
- 3 tsp. lemon juice

Directions:
1. Grind the ingredients except for the egg and form a smooth paste. Coat the yam in the paste. Now, beat the eggs and add a little salt to it.
2. Dip the coated vegetables in the egg mixture and then transfer to the sesame seeds and coat the yam well. Place the vegetables on a stick.
3. Pre heat the oven at 160 degrees Fahrenheit for around 5 minutes. Place the sticks in the basket and let them cook for another 25 minutes at the same temperature. Turn the sticks over in between the cooking process to get a uniform cook.

435.Vegetable Skewer

Ingredients:
- 3 tbsp. cream
- 3 eggs
- 2 cups mixed vegetables
- 3 onions chopped
- 5 green chilies
- 1 ½ tbsp. ginger paste
- 1 ½ tsp. garlic paste
- 1 ½ tsp. salt
- 2 ½ tbsp. white sesame seeds

Directions:
1. Grind the ingredients except for the egg and form a smooth paste. Coat the vegetables in the paste. Now, beat the eggs and add a little salt to it.
2. Dip the coated vegetables in the egg mixture and then transfer to the sesame seeds and coat the vegetables well. Place the vegetables on a stick.
3. Pre heat the oven at 160 degrees Fahrenheit for around 5 minutes. Place the sticks in the basket and let them cook for another 25 minutes at the same temperature. Turn the sticks over in between the cooking process to get a uniform cook.

436.Potato Club Barbeque Sandwich

Ingredients:
- ½ flake garlic crushed
- ¼ cup chopped onion
- ¼ tbsp. red chili sauce
- 2 slices of white bread
- 1 tbsp. softened butter
- 1 cup boiled potato
- 1 small capsicum
- ¼ tbsp. Worcestershire sauce
- ½ tsp. olive oil

Directions:
1. Take the slices of bread and remove the edges. Now cut the slices horizontally.
2. Cook the ingredients for the sauce and wait till it thickens. Now, add the potato to the sauce and stir till it obtains the flavors. Roast the capsicum and peel the skin off. Cut the capsicum into slices. Mix the ingredients together and apply it to the bread slices.
3. Pre-heat the oven for 5 minutes at 300 Fahrenheit. Open the basket of the Fryer and place the prepared Classic Sandwiches in it such that no two Classic Sandwiches are touching each other. Now keep the fryer at 250 degrees for around 15 minutes. Turn the Classic Sandwiches in between the cooking process to cook both slices. Serve the Classic Sandwiches with tomato ketchup or mint sauce.

437.Teriyaki Tofu

Servings: 3
Cooking Time: 15 Minutes
Ingredients:
- Nonstick cooking spray
- 14 oz. firm or extra firm tofu, pressed & cut in 1-inch cubes
- ¼ cup cornstarch
- ½ tsp salt
- ½ tsp ginger
- ½ tsp white pepper
- 3 tbsp. olive oil
- 12 oz. bottle vegan teriyaki sauce

Directions:
1. Lightly spray baking pan with cooking spray.
2. In a shallow dish, combine cornstarch, salt, ginger, and pepper.
3. Heat oil in a large skillet over med-high heat.
4. Toss tofu cubes in cornstarch mixture then add to skillet. Cook 5 minutes, turning over halfway through, until tofu is nicely seared. Transfer the tofu to the prepared baking pan.
5. Set oven to convection bake on 350°F for 15 minutes.
6. Pour all but ½ cup teriyaki sauce over tofu and stir to coat. After oven has preheated for 5 minutes,

place the baking pan in position 2 and bake tofu 10 minutes.

7.   Turn tofu over, spoon the sauce in the pan over it and bake another 10 minutes. Serve with reserved sauce for dipping.

Nutrition Info: Calories 469, Total Fat 25g, Saturated Fat 4g, Total Carbs 33g, Net Carbs 30g, Protein 28g, Sugar 16g, Fiber 3g, Sodium 2424mg, Potassium 571mg, Phosphorus 428mg

438.Chili Sweet Potato Fries

Servings: 4
Cooking Time: 30 Minutes
Ingredients:
- ½ tsp salt
- ½ tsp garlic powder
- ½ tsp chili powder
- ¼ tsp ground cumin
- 3 tbsp olive oil
- 3 sweet potatoes, cut into thick strips

Directions:
1.   In a bowl, mix salt, garlic powder, chili powder, and cumin, and whisk in oil. Coat in the potato strips and arrange them on the basket, without overcrowding. Press Start and cook for 20-25 minutes at 380 F on AirFry function or until crispy. Serve hot.

439.Beetroot Chips

Servings: 3
Cooking Time: 25 Minutes
Ingredients:
- 1lb golden beetroots, sliced
- 2 tbsp olive oil
- 1 tbsp yeast flakes
- 1 tsp vegan seasoning
- Salt to taste

Directions:
1.   In a bowl, add the olive oil, beetroots, vegan seasoning, and yeast and mix well. Dump the coated chips in the basket.
2.   Fit in the baking tray and cook in your for 15 minutes at 370 F on Air Fry function, shaking once halfway through. Serve.

440.Burger Cutlet

Ingredients:
- 1 tbsp. fresh coriander leaves. Chop them finely
- ¼ tsp. red chili powder
- ½ cup of boiled peas
- ¼ tsp. cumin powder
- 1 large potato boiled and mashed

- ½ cup breadcrumbs
- A pinch of salt to taste
- ¼ tsp. ginger finely chopped
- 1 green chili finely chopped
- 1 tsp. lemon juice
- ¼ tsp. dried mango powder

Directions:
1.   Mix the ingredients together and ensure that the flavors are right. You will now make round cutlets with the mixture and roll them out well.
2.   Pre heat the oven at 250 Fahrenheit for 5 minutes. Open the basket of the Fryer and arrange the cutlets in the basket. Close it carefully. Keep the fryer at 150 degrees for around 10 or 12 minutes. In between the cooking process, turn the cutlets over to get a uniform cook. Serve hot with mint sauce.

441.Cheesy Asparagus And Potato Platter

Servings: 5
Cooking Time: 26 Minutes
Ingredients:
- 4 medium potatoes, cut into wedges
- Cooking spray
- 1 bunch asparagus, trimmed
- 2 tablespoons olive oil
- Salt and pepper, to taste
- Cheese Sauce:
- ¼ cup crumbled cottage cheese
- ¼ cup buttermilk
- 1 tablespoon whole-grain mustard
- Salt and black pepper, to taste

Directions:
1.   Spritz the air fryer basket with cooking spray.
2.   Put the potatoes in the air fryer basket.
3.   Put the air fryer basket on the baking pan and slide into Rack Position 2, select Roast, set temperature to 400ºF (205ºC) and set time to 20 minutes.
4.   Stir the potatoes halfway through.
5.   When cooking is complete, the potatoes should be golden brown.
6.   Remove the potatoes from the oven to a platter. Cover the potatoes with foil to keep warm. Set aside.
7.   Place the asparagus in the air fryer basket and drizzle with the olive oil. Sprinkle with salt and pepper.
8.   Put the air fryer basket on the baking pan and slide into Rack Position 2, select Roast, set temperature to 400ºF (205ºC) and set time to 6 minutes. Stir the asparagus halfway through.
9.   When cooking is complete, the asparagus should be crispy.
10.   Meanwhile, make the cheese sauce by stirring together the cottage cheese, buttermilk, and mustard

in a small bowl. Season as needed with salt and pepper.

11.   Transfer the asparagus to the platter of potatoes and drizzle with the cheese sauce. Serve immediately.

442.Pumpkin French Cuisine Galette

Ingredients:
- 2 or 3 green chilies finely chopped
- 1 ½ tbsp. lemon juice
- Salt and pepper to taste
- 2 tbsp. garam masala
- 1 cup sliced pumpkin
- 3 tsp. ginger finely chopped
- 1-2 tbsp. fresh coriander leaves

Directions:
1.   Mix the ingredients in a clean bowl.
2.   Mold this mixture into round and flat French Cuisine Galettes.
3.   Wet the French Cuisine Galettes slightly with water.
4.   Pre heat the oven at 160 degrees Fahrenheit for 5 minutes. Place the French Cuisine Galettes in the fry basket and let them cook for another 25 minutes at the same temperature. Keep rolling them over to get a uniform cook. Serve either with mint sauce or ketchup.

443.Mom's Blooming Buttery Onion

Servings: 4
Cooking Time: 40 Minutes
Ingredients:
- 4 onions
- 2 tbsp butter, melted
- 1 tbsp olive oil

Directions:
1.   Preheat on Air Fry function to 350 F. Peel the onions and slice off the root bottom so it can sit well. Cut slices into the onion to make it look like a blooming flower, make sure not to go all the way through; four cuts will do.
2.   Place the onions in a greased baking tray. Drizzle with olive oil and butter and cook for about 30 minutes. Serve with garlic mayo dip.

444.Easy Cheesy Vegetable Quesadilla

Servings: 1
Cooking Time: 10 Minutes
Ingredients:
- 1 teaspoon olive oil
- 2 flour tortillas
- ¼ zucchini, sliced
- ¼ yellow bell pepper, sliced
- ¼ cup shredded gouda cheese
- 1 tablespoon chopped cilantro
- ½ green onion, sliced

Directions:
1.   Coat the air fryer basket with 1 teaspoon of olive oil.
2.   Arrange a flour tortilla in the basket and scatter the top with zucchini, bell pepper, gouda cheese, cilantro, and green onion. Place the other flour tortilla on top.
3.   Put the air fryer basket on the baking pan and slide into Rack Position 2, select Air Fry, set temperature to 390ºF (199ºC), and set time to 10 minutes.
4.   When cooking is complete, the tortillas should be lightly browned and the vegetables should be tender. Remove from the oven and cool for 5 minutes before slicing into wedges.

445.Balsamic Eggplant Caviar

Servings: 4
Cooking Time: 20 Minutes
Ingredients:
- 3 medium eggplants
- ½ red onion, chopped and blended
- 2 tbsp balsamic vinegar
- 1 tbsp olive oil
- Salt to taste

Directions:
1.   Arrange the eggplants on the basket and cook them in the Breville oven for 15 minutes at 380 F on Bake function. Let cool. Cut the eggplants in half, lengthwise and empty their insides.
2.   Pulse the onion the inside of the eggplants in a blender. Add in vinegar, olive oil, and salt, then blend again. Serve cool with bread and tomato sauce or ketchup.

446.Sweet-and-sour Brussels Sprouts

Servings: 2
Cooking Time: 20 Minutes
Ingredients:
- ¼ cup Thai sweet chili sauce
- 2 tablespoons black vinegar or balsamic vinegar
- ½ teaspoon hot sauce
- 2 small shallots, cut into ¼-inch-thick slices
- 8 ounces (227 g) Brussels sprouts, trimmed (large sprouts halved)
- Kosher salt and freshly ground black pepper, to taste
- 2 teaspoons lightly packed fresh cilantro leaves, for garnish

Directions:

1. Place the chili sauce, vinegar, and hot sauce in a large bowl and whisk to combine.
2. Add the shallots and Brussels sprouts and toss to coat. Sprinkle with the salt and pepper. Transfer the Brussels sprouts and sauce to the baking pan.
3. Slide the baking pan into Rack Position 2, select Roast, set temperature to 390ºF (199ºC), and set time to 20 minutes.
4. Stir the Brussels sprouts twice during cooking.
5. When cooking is complete, the Brussels sprouts should be crisp-tender. Remove from the oven. Sprinkle the cilantro on top for garnish and serve warm.

447.Cheesy Cauliflower Fritters

Servings: 8
Cooking Time: 7 Minutes
Ingredients:
- ½ C. chopped parsley
- 1 C. Italian breadcrumbs
- 1/3 C. shredded mozzarella cheese
- 1/3 C. shredded sharp cheddar cheese
- 1 egg
- 2 minced garlic cloves
- 3 chopped scallions
- 1 head of cauliflower

Directions:
1. Preparing the Ingredients. Cut the cauliflower up into florets. Wash well and pat dry. Place into a food processor and pulse 20-30 seconds till it looks like rice.
2. Place cauliflower rice in a bowl and mix with pepper, salt, egg, cheeses, breadcrumbs, garlic, and scallions.
3. With hands, form 15 patties of the mixture. Add more breadcrumbs if needed.
4. Air Frying. With olive oil, spritz patties, and place into your air fryer oven in a single layer. Set temperature to 390°F, and set time to 7 minutes, flipping after 7 minutes.
Nutrition Info: CALORIES: 209; FAT: 17G; PROTEIN: 6G; SUGAR:0.5

448.Broccoli Momo's Recipe

Ingredients:
- 2 tbsp. oil
- 2 tsp. ginger-garlic paste
- 2 tsp. soya sauce
- 2 tsp. vinegar
- 1 ½ cup all-purpose flour
- ½ tsp. salt
- 5 tbsp. water
- 2 cups grated broccoli

Directions:
1. Squeeze the dough and cover it with plastic wrap and set aside. Next, cook the ingredients for the filling and try to ensure that the broccoli is covered well with the sauce.
2. Roll the dough and cut it into a square. Place the filling in the center. Now, wrap the dough to cover the filling and pinch the edges together.
3. Pre heat the oven at 200° F for 5 minutes. Place the gnocchi's in the fry basket and close it. Let them cook at the same temperature for another 20 minutes. Recommended sides are chili sauce or ketchup.

449.Cayenne Spicy Green Beans

Servings: 4
Cooking Time: 20 Minutes
Ingredients:
- 1 cup panko breadcrumbs
- 2 whole eggs, beaten
- ½ cup Parmesan cheese, grated
- ½ cup flour
- 1 tsp cayenne pepper
- 1 ½ pounds green beans
- Salt to taste

Directions:
1. In a bowl, mix panko breadcrumbs, Parmesan cheese, cayenne pepper, salt, and pepper. Roll the green beans in flour and dip in eggs. Dredge beans in the parmesan-panko mix. Place the prepared beans in the greased cooking basket and fit in the baking tray; cook for 15 minutes on Air Fry function at 350 F, shaking once. Serve and enjoy!

450.Rosemary Squash With Cheese

Servings: 2
Cooking Time: 20 Minutes
Ingredients:
- 1 pound (454 g) butternut squash, cut into wedges
- 2 tablespoons olive oil
- 1 tablespoon dried rosemary
- Salt, to salt
- 1 cup crumbled goat cheese
- 1 tablespoon maple syrup

Directions:
1. Toss the squash wedges with the olive oil, rosemary, and salt in a large bowl until well coated.
2. Transfer the squash wedges to the air fryer basket, spreading them out in as even a layer as possible.
3. Put the air fryer basket on the baking pan and slide into Rack Position 2, select Air Fry, set

temperature to 350ºF (180ºC), and set time to 20 minutes.

4.   After 10 minutes, remove from the oven and flip the squash. Return the pan to the oven and continue cooking for 10 minutes.

5.   When cooking is complete, the squash should be golden brown. Remove from the oven. Sprinkle the goat cheese on top and serve drizzled with the maple syrup.

451.Roasted Vegetables With Basil

Servings: 2
Cooking Time: 20 Minutes
Ingredients:
- 1 small eggplant, halved and sliced
- 1 yellow bell pepper, cut into thick strips
- 1 red bell pepper, cut into thick strips
- 2 garlic cloves, quartered
- 1 red onion, sliced
- 1 tablespoon extra-virgin olive oil
- Salt and freshly ground black pepper, to taste
- ½ cup chopped fresh basil, for garnish
- Cooking spray

Directions:
1.   Grease the baking pan with cooking spray.
2.   Place the eggplant, bell peppers, garlic, and red onion in the greased baking pan. Drizzle with the olive oil and toss to coat well. Spritz any uncoated surfaces with cooking spray.
3.   Slide the baking pan into Rack Position 1, select Convection Bake, set temperature to 350ºF (180ºC), and set time to 20 minutes.
4.   Flip the vegetables halfway through the cooking time.
5.   When done, remove from the oven and sprinkle with salt and pepper.
6.   Sprinkle the basil on top for garnish and serve.

452.Coconut Vegan Fries

Servings: 2
Cooking Time: 20 Minutes
Ingredients:
- 2 potatoes, spiralized
- 1 tbsp tomato ketchup
- 2 tbsp olive oil
- Salt and black pepper to taste
- 2 tbsp coconut oil

Directions:
1.   In a bowl, mix olive oil, coconut oil, salt, and pepper. Add in the potatoes and toss to coat. Place them in the basket and fit in the baking tray; cook for 15 minutes on Air Fry function at 360 F. Serve with ketchup and enjoy!

453.Okra Flat Cakes

Ingredients:
- 2 or 3 green chilies finely chopped
- 1 ½ tbsp. lemon juice
- Salt and pepper to taste
- 2 tbsp. garam masala
- 2 cups sliced okra
- 3 tsp. ginger finely chopped
- 1-2 tbsp. fresh coriander leaves

Directions:
1.   Mix the ingredients in a clean bowl and add water to it. Make sure that the
2.   paste is not too watery but is enough to apply on the okra.
3.   Pre heat the oven at 160 degrees Fahrenheit for 5 minutes. Place the French Cuisine Galettes in the fry basket and let them cook for another 25 minutes at the same temperature. Keep rolling them over to get a uniform cook. Serve either with mint sauce or ketchup.

454.Onion French Cuisine Galette

Ingredients:
- 2 or 3 green chilies finely chopped
- 1 ½ tbsp. lemon juice
- Salt and pepper to taste
- 2 tbsp. garam masala
- 2 medium onions (Cut long)
- 1 ½ cup coarsely crushed peanuts
- 3 tsp. ginger finely chopped
- 1-2 tbsp. fresh coriander leaves

Directions:
1.   Mix the ingredients in a clean bowl.
2.   Mold this mixture into round and flat French Cuisine Galettes.
3.   Wet the French Cuisine Galettes slightly with water. Coat each French Cuisine Galette with the crushed peanuts.
4.   Pre heat the oven at 160 degrees Fahrenheit for 5 minutes. Place the French Cuisine Galettes in the fry basket and let them cook for another 25 minutes at the same temperature. Keep rolling them over to get a uniform cook. Serve either with mint sauce or ketchup.

455.Cottage Cheese And Mushroom Mexican Burritos

Ingredients:
- ½ cup mushrooms thinly sliced

- 1 cup cottage cheese cut in too long and slightly thick Oregano Fingers
- A pinch of salt to taste
- ½ tsp. red chili flakes
- 1 tsp. freshly ground peppercorns
- ½ cup pickled jalapenos
- 1-2 lettuce leaves shredded.
- ½ cup red kidney beans (soaked overnight)
- ½ small onion chopped
- 1 tbsp. olive oil
- 2 tbsp. tomato puree
- ¼ tsp. red chili powder
- 1 tsp. of salt to taste
- 4-5 flour tortillas
- 1 or 2 spring onions chopped finely. Also cut the greens.
- Take one tomato. Remove the seeds and chop it into small pieces.
- 1 green chili chopped.
- 1 cup of cheddar cheese grated.
- 1 cup boiled rice (not necessary).
- A few flour tortillas to put the filing in.

Directions:
1. Cook the beans along with the onion and garlic and mash them finely.
2. Now, make the sauce you will need for the burrito. Ensure that you create a slightly thick sauce.
3. For the filling, you will need to cook the ingredients well in a pan and ensure that the vegetables have browned on the outside.
4. To make the salad, toss the ingredients together. Place the tortilla and add a layer of sauce, followed by the beans and the filling at the center. Before you roll it, you will need to place the salad on top of the filling.
5. Pre-heat the oven for around 5 minutes at 200 Fahrenheit. Open the fry basket and keep the burritos inside. Close the basket properly. Let the Air
6. Fryer remain at 200 Fahrenheit for another 15 minutes or so. Halfway through, remove the basket and turn all the burritos over in order to get a uniform cook.

456.Bitter Gourd Flat Cakes

Ingredients:
- 2 or 3 green chilies finely chopped
- 1 ½ tbsp. lemon juice
- Salt and pepper to taste
- 2 tbsp. garam masala
- 2 cups sliced bitter gourd
- 3 tsp. ginger finely chopped
- 1-2 tbsp. fresh coriander leaves

Directions:
1. Mix the ingredients in a clean bowl and add water to it. Make sure that the paste is not too watery but is enough to apply on the bitter gourd slices.
2. Pre heat the oven at 160 degrees Fahrenheit for 5 minutes. Place the French Cuisine Galettes in the fry basket and let them cook for another 25 minutes at the same temperature. Keep rolling them over to get a uniform cook. Serve either with mint sauce or ketchup.

OTHER FAVORITE RECIPES

457.Crunchy Green Tomatoes Slices

Servings: 12 Slices
Cooking Time: 8 Minutes
Ingredients:
- ½ cup all-purpose flour
- 1 egg
- ½ cup buttermilk
- 1 cup cornmeal
- 1 cup panko
- 2 green tomatoes, cut into ¼-inch-thick slices, patted dry
- ½ teaspoon salt
- ½ teaspoon ground black pepper
- Cooking spray

Directions:
1. Spritz a baking sheet with cooking spray.
2. Pour the flour in a bowl. Whisk the egg and buttermilk in a second bowl. Combine the cornmeal and panko in a third bowl.
3. Dredge the tomato slices in the bowl of flour first, then into the egg mixture, and then dunk the slices into the cornmeal mixture. Shake the excess off.
4. Transfer the well-coated tomato slices in the baking sheet and sprinkle with salt and ground black pepper. Spritz the tomato slices with cooking spray.
5. Put the air fryer basket on the baking pan and slide into Rack Position 2, select Air Fry, set temperature to 400ºF (205ºC) and set time to 8 minutes.
6. Flip the slices halfway through the cooking time.
7. When cooking is complete, the tomato slices should be crispy and lightly browned. Remove the baking sheet from the oven.
8. Serve immediately.

458.Chorizo, Corn, And Potato Frittata

Servings: 4
Cooking Time: 12 Minutes
Ingredients:
- 2 tablespoons olive oil
- 1 chorizo, sliced
- 4 eggs
- ½ cup corn
- 1 large potato, boiled and cubed
- 1 tablespoon chopped parsley
- ½ cup feta cheese, crumbled
- Salt and ground black pepper, to taste

Directions:
1. Heat the olive oil in a nonstick skillet over medium heat until shimmering.
2. Add the chorizo and cook for 4 minutes or until golden brown.
3. Whisk the eggs in a bowl, then sprinkle with salt and ground black pepper.
4. Mix the remaining ingredients in the egg mixture, then pour the chorizo and its fat into the baking pan. Pour in the egg mixture.
5. Slide the baking pan into Rack Position 1, select Convection Bake, set temperature to 330ºF (166ºC) and set time to 8 minutes.
6. Stir the mixture halfway through.
7. When cooking is complete, the eggs should be set.
8. Serve immediately.

459.Dehydrated Honey-rosemary Roasted Almonds

Ingredients:
- 1 heaping tablespoon demerara sugar
- 1 teaspoon finely chopped fresh rosemary
- 1 teaspoon kosher salt
- 8 ounces (225g) raw almonds
- 2 tablespoons kosher salt
- Honey-Rosemary glaze
- ¼ cup (80g) honey

Directions:
1. Place almonds and salt in a bowl. Add cold tap water to cover the almonds by 1-inch
2. (2cm). Let soak at room temperature for 12 hours to activate.
3. Rinse almonds under cold running water, then drain. Spread in a single layer on the dehydrate basket.
4. Dehydrate almonds for 24 hours or till tender and somewhat crispy but additionally spongy in the middle. Almonds may be eaten plain or roasted each the next recipe.
5. Put honey in a small saucepan and heat over Low heat. Put triggered nuts
6. At a medium bowl and then pour over warm honey. Stir To coat nuts equally. Add rosemary, sugar
7. And salt and stir to blend.
8. Spread Almonds in one layer on the skillet.
9. Insert cable rack into rack place 6. Select BAKE/350°F (175°C)/CONVECTION/10 moments and empower Rotate Remind.
10. Stirring almonds when Rotate Remind signs.
11. Let cool completely before storing in an airtight container.

460.Kale Chips With Soy Sauce

Servings: 2
Cooking Time: 5 Minutes
Ingredients:

- 4 medium kale leaves, about 1 ounce (28 g) each, stems removed, tear the leaves in thirds
- 2 teaspoons soy sauce
- 2 teaspoons olive oil

Directions:
1. Toss the kale leaves with soy sauce and olive oil in a large bowl to coat well. Place the leaves in the baking pan.
2. Put the air fryer basket on the baking pan and slide into Rack Position 2, select Air Fry, set temperature to 400ºF (205ºC) and set time to 5 minutes.
3. Flip the leaves with tongs gently halfway through.
4. When cooked, the kale leaves should be crispy. Remove from the oven and serve immediately.

461.Chicken Sausage And Broccoli Casserole

Servings: 8
Cooking Time: 20 Minutes
Ingredients:
- 10 eggs
- 1 cup Cheddar cheese, shredded and divided
- ¾ cup heavy whipping cream
- 1 (12-ounce / 340-g) package cooked chicken sausage
- 1 cup broccoli, chopped
- 2 cloves garlic, minced
- ½ tablespoon salt
- ¼ tablespoon ground black pepper
- Cooking spray

Directions:
1. Spritz the baking pan with cooking spray.
2. Whisk the eggs with Cheddar and cream in a large bowl to mix well.
3. Combine the cooked sausage, broccoli, garlic, salt, and ground black pepper in a separate bowl. Stir to mix well.
4. Pour the sausage mixture into the baking pan, then spread the egg mixture over to cover.
5. Slide the baking pan into Rack Position 1, select Convection Bake, set temperature to 400ºF (205ºC) and set time to 20 minutes.
6. When cooking is complete, the egg should be set and a toothpick inserted in the center should come out clean.
7. Serve immediately.

462.Lemony Shishito Peppers

Servings: 4
Cooking Time: 5 Minutes
Ingredients:

- ½ pound (227 g) shishito peppers (about 24)
- 1 tablespoon olive oil
- Coarse sea salt, to taste
- Lemon wedges, for serving
- Cooking spray

Directions:
1. Spritz the air fryer basket with cooking spray.
2. Toss the peppers with olive oil in a large bowl to coat well.
3. Arrange the peppers in the basket.
4. Put the air fryer basket on the baking pan and slide into Rack Position 2, select Air Fry, set temperature to 400ºF (205ºC) and set time to 5 minutes.
5. Flip the peppers and sprinkle the peppers with salt halfway through the cooking time.
6. When cooked, the peppers should be blistered and lightly charred. Transfer the peppers onto a plate and squeeze the lemon wedges on top before serving.

463.Crispy Cheese Wafer

Servings: 2
Cooking Time: 5 Minutes
Ingredients:
- 1 cup shredded aged Manchego cheese
- 1 teaspoon all-purpose flour
- ½ teaspoon cumin seeds
- ¼ teaspoon cracked black pepper

Directions:
1. Line the air fryer basket with parchment paper.
2. Combine the cheese and flour in a bowl. Stir to mix well. Spread the mixture in the pan into a 4-inch round.
3. Combine the cumin and black pepper in a small bowl. Stir to mix well. Sprinkle the cumin mixture over the cheese round.
4. Put the air fryer basket on the baking pan and slide into Rack Position 2, select Air Fry, set temperature to 375ºF (190ºC) and set time to 5 minutes.
5. When cooked, the cheese will be lightly browned and frothy.
6. Use tongs to transfer the cheese wafer onto a plate and slice to serve.

464.Apple Fritters With Sugary Glaze

Servings: 15 Fritters
Cooking Time: 8 Minutes
Ingredients:
- Apple Fritters:
- 2 firm apples, peeled, cored, and diced
- ½ teaspoon cinnamon
- Juice of 1 lemon

- 1 cup all-purpose flour
- 1½ teaspoons baking powder
- ½ teaspoon kosher salt
- 2 eggs
- ¼ cup milk
- 2 tablespoons unsalted butter, melted
- 2 tablespoons granulated sugar
- Cooking spray
- Glaze:
- ½ teaspoon vanilla extract
- 1¼ cups powdered sugar, sifted
- ¼ cup water

Directions:
1. Line the air fryer basket with parchment paper.
2. Combine the apples with cinnamon and lemon juice in a small bowl. Toss to coat well.
3. Combine the flour, baking powder, and salt in a large bowl. Stir to mix well.
4. Whisk the egg, milk, butter, and sugar in a medium bowl. Stir to mix well.
5. Make a well in the center of the flour mixture, then pour the egg mixture into the well and stir to mix well. Mix in the apple until a dough forms.
6. Use an ice cream scoop to scoop 15 balls from the dough onto the pan. Spritz with cooking spray.
7. Put the air fryer basket on the baking pan and slide into Rack Position 2, select Air Fry, set temperature to 360ºF (182ºC) and set time to 8 minutes.
8. Flip the apple fritters halfway through the cooking time.
9. Meanwhile, combine the ingredients for the glaze in a separate small bowl. Stir to mix well.
10. When cooking is complete, the apple fritters will be golden brown. Serve the fritters with the glaze on top or use the glaze for dipping.

465.Spicy Air Fried Old Bay Shrimp

Servings: 2 Cups
Cooking Time: 10 Minutes
Ingredients:
- ½ teaspoon Old Bay Seasoning
- 1 teaspoon ground cayenne pepper
- ½ teaspoon paprika
- 1 tablespoon olive oil
- ⅛ teaspoon salt
- ½ pound (227 g) shrimps, peeled and deveined
- Juice of half a lemon

Directions:
1. Combine the Old Bay Seasoning, cayenne pepper, paprika, olive oil, and salt in a large bowl, then add the shrimps and toss to coat well.
2. Put the shrimps in the air fryer basket.
3. Put the air fryer basket on the baking pan and slide into Rack Position 2, select Air Fry, set

temperature to 390ºF (199ºC) and set time to 10 minutes.
4. Flip the shrimps halfway through the cooking time.
5. When cooking is complete, the shrimps should be opaque. Serve the shrimps with lemon juice on top.

466.Smoked Trout And Crème Fraiche Frittata

Servings: 4
Cooking Time: 17 Minutes
Ingredients:
- 2 tablespoons olive oil
- 1 onion, sliced
- 1 egg, beaten
- ½ tablespoon horseradish sauce
- 6 tablespoons crème fraiche
- 1 cup diced smoked trout
- 2 tablespoons chopped fresh dill
- Cooking spray

Directions:
1. Spritz the baking pan with cooking spray.
2. Heat the olive oil in a nonstick skillet over medium heat until shimmering.
3. Add the onion and sauté for 3 minutes or until translucent.
4. Combine the egg, horseradish sauce, and crème fraiche in a large bowl. Stir to mix well, then mix in the sautéed onion, smoked trout, and dill.
5. Pour the mixture in the prepared baking pan.
6. Slide the baking pan into Rack Position 1, select Convection Bake, set temperature to 350ºF (180ºC) and set time to 14 minutes.
7. Stir the mixture halfway through.
8. When cooking is complete, the egg should be set and the edges should be lightly browned.
9. Serve immediately.

467.Burgundy Beef And Mushroom Casserole

Servings: 4
Cooking Time: 25 Minutes
Ingredients:
- 1½ pounds (680 g) beef steak
- 1 ounce (28 g) dry onion soup mix
- 2 cups sliced mushrooms
- 1 (14.5-ounce / 411-g) can cream of mushroom soup
- ½ cup beef broth
- ¼ cup red wine
- 3 garlic cloves, minced
- 1 whole onion, chopped

Directions:

1. Put the beef steak in a large bowl, then sprinkle with dry onion soup mix. Toss to coat well.
2. Combine the mushrooms with mushroom soup, beef broth, red wine, garlic, and onion in a large bowl. Stir to mix well.
3. Transfer the beef steak in the baking pan, then pour in the mushroom mixture.
4. Slide the baking pan into Rack Position 1, select Convection Bake, set temperature to 360ºF (182ºC) and set time to 25 minutes.
5. When cooking is complete, the mushrooms should be soft and the beef should be well browned.
6. Remove from the oven and serve immediately.

468.Herbed Cheddar Frittata

Servings: 4
Cooking Time: 20 Minutes
Ingredients:
- ½ cup shredded Cheddar cheese
- ½ cup half-and-half
- 4 large eggs
- 2 tablespoons chopped scallion greens
- 2 tablespoons chopped fresh parsley
- ½ teaspoon kosher salt
- ½ teaspoon ground black pepper
- Cooking spray

Directions:
1. Spritz the baking pan with cooking spray.
2. Whisk together all the ingredients in a large bowl, then pour the mixture into the prepared baking pan.
3. Slide the baking pan into Rack Position 1, select Convection Bake, set temperature to 300ºF (150ºC) and set time to 20 minutes.
4. Stir the mixture halfway through.
5. When cooking is complete, the eggs should be set.
6. Serve immediately.

469.Cinnamon Rolls With Cream Glaze

Servings: 8
Cooking Time: 5 Minutes
Ingredients:
- 1 pound (454 g) frozen bread dough, thawed
- 2 tablespoons melted butter
- 1½ tablespoons cinnamon
- ¾ cup brown sugar
- Cooking spray
- Cream Glaze:
- 4 ounces (113 g) softened cream cheese
- ½ teaspoon vanilla extract
- 2 tablespoons melted butter
- 1¼ cups powdered erythritol

Directions:
1. Place the bread dough on a clean work surface, then roll the dough out into a rectangle with a rolling pin.
2. Brush the top of the dough with melted butter and leave 1-inch edges uncovered.
3. Combine the cinnamon and sugar in a small bowl, then sprinkle the dough with the cinnamon mixture.
4. Roll the dough over tightly, then cut the dough log into 8 portions. Wrap the portions in plastic, better separately, and let sit to rise for 1 or 2 hours.
5. Meanwhile, combine the ingredients for the glaze in a separate small bowl. Stir to mix well.
6. Spritz the air fryer basket with cooking spray. Transfer the risen rolls to the basket.
7. Put the air fryer basket on the baking pan and slide into Rack Position 2, select Air Fry, set temperature to 350ºF (180ºC) and set time to 5 minutes.
8. Flip the rolls halfway through the cooking time.
9. When cooking is complete, the rolls will be golden brown.
10. Serve the rolls with the glaze.

470.Ritzy Pimento And Almond Turkey Casserole

Servings: 4
Cooking Time: 32 Minutes
Ingredients:
- 1 pound (454 g) turkey breasts
- 1 tablespoon olive oil
- 2 boiled eggs, chopped
- 2 tablespoons chopped pimentos
- ¼ cup slivered almonds, chopped
- ¼ cup mayonnaise
- ½ cup diced celery
- 2 tablespoons chopped green onion
- ¼ cup cream of chicken soup
- ¼ cup bread crumbs
- Salt and ground black pepper, to taste

Directions:
1. Put the turkey breasts in a large bowl. Sprinkle with salt and ground black pepper and drizzle with olive oil. Toss to coat well.
2. Transfer the turkey to the air fryer basket.
3. Put the air fryer basket on the baking pan and slide into Rack Position 2, select Air Fry, set temperature to 390ºF (199ºC) and set time to 12 minutes.
4. Flip the turkey halfway through.
5. When cooking is complete, the turkey should be well browned.
6. Remove the turkey breasts from the oven and cut into cubes, then combine the chicken cubes with

eggs, pimentos, almonds, mayo, celery, green onions, and chicken soup in a large bowl. Stir to mix.
7. Pour the mixture into the baking pan, then spread with bread crumbs.
8. Slide the baking pan into Rack Position 1, select Convection Bake, set time to 20 minutes.
9. When cooking is complete, the eggs should be set.
10. Remove from the oven and serve immediately.

471.Mediterranean Quiche

Servings: 4
Cooking Time: 30 Minutes
Ingredients:
- 4 eggs
- ¼ cup chopped Kalamata olives
- ½ cup chopped tomatoes
- ¼ cup chopped onion
- ½ cup milk
- 1 cup crumbled feta cheese
- ½ tablespoon chopped oregano
- ½ tablespoon chopped basil
- Salt and ground black pepper, to taste
- Cooking spray

Directions:
1. Spritz the baking pan with cooking spray.
2. Whisk the eggs with remaining ingredients in a large bowl. Stir to mix well.
3. Pour the mixture into the prepared baking pan.
4. Slide the baking pan into Rack Position 1, select Convection Bake, set temperature to 340ºF (171ºC) and set time to 30 minutes.
5. When cooking is complete, the eggs should be set and a toothpick inserted in the center should come out clean.
6. Serve immediately.

472.Golden Salmon And Carrot Croquettes

Servings: 6
Cooking Time: 10 Minutes
Ingredients:
- 2 egg whites
- 1 cup almond flour
- 1 cup panko bread crumbs
- 1 pound (454 g) chopped salmon fillet
- $^2/_3$ cup grated carrots
- 2 tablespoons minced garlic cloves
- ½ cup chopped onion
- 2 tablespoons chopped chives
- Cooking spray

Directions:
1. Spritz the air fryer basket with cooking spray.

2. Whisk the egg whites in a bowl. Put the flour in a second bowl. Pour the bread crumbs in a third bowl. Set aside.
3. Combine the salmon, carrots, garlic, onion, and chives in a large bowl. Stir to mix well.
4. Form the mixture into balls with your hands. Dredge the balls into the flour, then egg, and then bread crumbs to coat well.
5. Arrange the salmon balls on the basket and spritz with cooking spray.
6. Put the air fryer basket on the baking pan and slide into Rack Position 2, select Air Fry, set temperature to 350ºF (180ºC) and set time to 10 minutes.
7. Flip the salmon balls halfway through cooking.
8. When cooking is complete, the salmon balls will be crispy and browned. Remove from the oven and serve immediately.

473.Chicken Divan

Servings: 4
Cooking Time: 24 Minutes
Ingredients:
- 4 chicken breasts
- Salt and ground black pepper, to taste
- 1 head broccoli, cut into florets
- ½ cup cream of mushroom soup
- 1 cup shredded Cheddar cheese
- ½ cup croutons
- Cooking spray

Directions:
1. Spritz the air fryer basket with cooking spray.
2. Put the chicken breasts in the basket and sprinkle with salt and ground black pepper.
3. Put the air fryer basket on the baking pan and slide into Rack Position 2, select Air Fry, set temperature to 390ºF (199ºC) and set time to 14 minutes.
4. Flip the breasts halfway through the cooking time.
5. When cooking is complete, the breasts should be well browned and tender.
6. Remove the breasts from the oven and allow to cool for a few minutes on a plate, then cut the breasts into bite-size pieces.
7. Combine the chicken, broccoli, mushroom soup, and Cheddar cheese in a large bowl. Stir to mix well.
8. Spritz the baking pan with cooking spray. Pour the chicken mixture into the pan. Spread the croutons over the mixture.
9. Slide the baking pan into Rack Position 1, select Convection Bake, set time to 10 minutes.
10. When cooking is complete, the croutons should be lightly browned and the mixture should be set.
11. Remove from the oven and serve immediately.

474.Air Fried Crispy Brussels Sprouts

Servings: 4
Cooking Time: 20 Minutes
Ingredients:
- ¼ teaspoon salt
- ⅛ teaspoon ground black pepper
- 1 tablespoon extra-virgin olive oil
- 1 pound (454 g) Brussels sprouts, trimmed and halved
- Lemon wedges, for garnish

Directions:
1. Combine the salt, black pepper, and olive oil in a large bowl. Stir to mix well.
2. Add the Brussels sprouts to the bowl of mixture and toss to coat well. Arrange the Brussels sprouts in the air fryer basket.
3. Put the air fryer basket on the baking pan and slide into Rack Position 2, select Air Fry, set temperature to 350ºF (180ºC) and set time to 20 minutes.
4. Stir the Brussels sprouts two times during cooking.
5. When cooked, the Brussels sprouts will be lightly browned and wilted. Transfer the cooked Brussels sprouts to a large plate and squeeze the lemon wedges on top to serve.

475.Chocolate Buttermilk Cake

Servings: 8
Cooking Time: 20 Minutes
Ingredients:
- 1 cup all-purpose flour
- ⅔ cup granulated white sugar
- ¼ cup unsweetened cocoa powder
- ¾ teaspoon baking soda
- ¼ teaspoon salt
- ⅔ cup buttermilk
- 2 tablespoons plus 2 teaspoons vegetable oil
- 1 teaspoon vanilla extract
- Cooking spray

Directions:
1. Spritz the baking pan with cooking spray.
2. Combine the flour, cocoa powder, baking soda, sugar, and salt in a large bowl. Stir to mix well.
3. Mix in the buttermilk, vanilla, and vegetable oil. Keep stirring until it forms a grainy and thick dough.
4. Scrape the chocolate batter from the bowl and transfer to the pan, level the batter in an even layer with a spatula.
5. Slide the baking pan into Rack Position 1, select Convection Bake, set temperature to 325ºF (163ºC) and set time to 20 minutes.

6. After 15 minutes, remove the pan from the oven. Check the doneness. Return the pan to the oven and continue cooking.
7. When done, a toothpick inserted in the center should come out clean.
8. Invert the cake on a cooling rack and allow to cool for 15 minutes before slicing to serve.

476.Oven Baked Rice

Servings: About 4 Cups
Cooking Time: 35 Minutes
Ingredients:
- 1 cup long-grain white rice, rinsed and drained
- 1 tablespoon unsalted butter, melted, or 1 tablespoon extra-virgin olive oil
- 2 cups water
- 1 teaspoon kosher salt or ½ teaspoon fine salt

Directions:
1. Add the butter and rice to the baking pan and stir to coat. Pour in the water and sprinkle with the salt. Stir until the salt is dissolved.
2. Select Bake, set the temperature to 325ºF (163ºC), and set the time for 35 minutes. Select Start to begin preheating.
3. Once the unit has preheated, place the pan in the oven.
4. After 20 minutes, remove the pan from the oven. Stir the rice. Transfer the pan back to the oven and continue cooking for 10 to 15 minutes, or until the rice is mostly cooked through and the water is absorbed.
5. When done, remove the pan from the oven and cover with aluminum foil. Let stand for 10 minutes. Using a fork, gently fluff the rice.
6. Serve immediately.

477.Dehydrated Vegetable Black Pepper Chips

Ingredients:
- Spice mix for parsnip chips
- ½ teaspoon ground turmeric
- 1 teaspoon kosher salt
- ½ teaspoon ground white or black pepper
- Red wine vinegar glaze for beet chips
- 2 tablespoons red wine vinegar
- 1 medium sweet potato
- 2 medium parsnips
- 2 medium beets
- Spice mix for sweet potato chips
- ½ teaspoon dried thyme
- ½ teaspoon onion powder
- ½ teaspoon garlic powder
- ¼ teaspoon ground white pepper

- 1 teaspoon kosher salt
- ½ teaspoon kosher salt
- ½ teaspoon ground white or black pepper

Directions:
1. For the sweet potato chips, combine spice mix in a little bowl and set aside. Peel sweet curry then slice using a mandolin.
2. Arrange slices in One coating on the dehydrate baskets. Gently and evenly sprinkle with the spice mixture. Place dehydrate baskets in rack positions 5 and 3 and press START. Assess on crispiness and rotate trays occasionally, every 4--5 hours.
3. Chips should sense paper-dry and snap in half easily. For the parsnip chips, combine spice mix in a little bowl and set aside. Arrange pieces in a single layer on the dehydrate baskets. Lightly and evenly sprinkle with the spice mixture.
4. Dehydrate chips as per step 3, altering the dehydrate period to 6 hours. For the beet chips, peel beets then thinly slice using a mandolin. Arrange slices in a single layer on the dehydrate baskets. Lightly brush with red wine vinegar then lightly and evenly sprinkle with pepper and salt. Dehydrate chips According to step 3.

478.Broccoli, Carrot, And Tomato Quiche

Servings: 4
Cooking Time: 14 Minutes
Ingredients:
- 4 eggs
- 1 teaspoon dried thyme
- 1 cup whole milk
- 1 steamed carrots, diced
- 2 cups steamed broccoli florets
- 2 medium tomatoes, diced
- ¼ cup crumbled feta cheese
- 1 cup grated Cheddar cheese
- 1 teaspoon chopped parsley
- Salt and ground black pepper, to taste
- Cooking spray

Directions:
1. Spritz the baking pan with cooking spray.
2. Whisk together the eggs, thyme, salt, and ground black pepper in a bowl and fold in the milk while mixing.
3. Put the carrots, broccoli, and tomatoes in the prepared baking pan, then spread with feta cheese and ½ cup Cheddar cheese. Pour the egg mixture over, then scatter with remaining Cheddar on top.
4. Slide the baking pan into Rack Position 1, select Convection Bake, set temperature to 350ºF (180ºC) and set time to 14 minutes.
5. When cooking is complete, the egg should be set and the quiche should be puffed.

6. Remove the quiche from the oven and top with chopped parsley, then slice to serve.

479.Simple Air Fried Edamame

Servings: 6
Cooking Time: 7 Minutes
Ingredients:
- 1½ pounds (680 g) unshelled edamame
- 2 tablespoons olive oil
- 1 teaspoon sea salt

Directions:
1. Place the edamame in a large bowl, then drizzle with olive oil. Toss to coat well. Transfer the edamame to the air fryer basket.
2. Put the air fryer basket on the baking pan and slide into Rack Position 2, select Air Fry, set temperature to 400ºF (205ºC) and set time to 7 minutes.
3. Stir the edamame at least three times during cooking.
4. When done, the edamame will be tender and warmed through.
5. Transfer the cooked edamame onto a plate and sprinkle with salt. Toss to combine well and set aside for 3 minutes to infuse before serving.

480.Simple Butter Cake

Servings: 8
Cooking Time: 20 Minutes
Ingredients:
- 1 cup all-purpose flour
- 1¼ teaspoons baking powder
- ¼ teaspoon salt
- ½ cup plus 1½ tablespoons granulated white sugar
- 9½ tablespoons butter, at room temperature
- 2 large eggs
- 1 large egg yolk
- 2½ tablespoons milk
- 1 teaspoon vanilla extract
- Cooking spray

Directions:
1. Spritz the baking pan with cooking spray.
2. Combine the flour, baking powder, and salt in a large bowl. Stir to mix well.
3. Whip the sugar and butter in a separate bowl with a hand mixer on medium speed for 3 minutes.
4. Whip the eggs, egg yolk, milk, and vanilla extract into the sugar and butter mix with a hand mixer.
5. Pour in the flour mixture and whip with hand mixer until sanity and smooth.
6. Scrape the batter into the baking pan and level the batter with a spatula.

7. Slide the baking pan into Rack Position 1, select Convection Bake, set temperature to 325ºF (163ºC) and set time to 20 minutes.
8. After 15 minutes, remove the pan from the oven. Check the doneness. Return the pan to the oven and continue cooking.
9. When done, a toothpick inserted in the center should come out clean.
10. Invert the cake on a cooling rack and allow to cool for 15 minutes before slicing to serve.

481.Classic Worcestershire Poutine

Servings: 2
Cooking Time: 33 Minutes
Ingredients:
- 2 russet potatoes, scrubbed and cut into ½-inch sticks
- 2 teaspoons vegetable oil
- 2 tablespoons butter
- ¼ onion, minced
- ¼ teaspoon dried thyme
- 1 clove garlic, smashed
- 3 tablespoons all-purpose flour
- 1 teaspoon tomato paste
- 1½ cups beef stock
- 2 teaspoons Worcestershire sauce
- Salt and freshly ground black pepper, to taste
- $^2/_3$ cup chopped string cheese

Directions:
1. Bring a pot of water to a boil, then put in the potato sticks and blanch for 4 minutes.
2. Drain the potato sticks and rinse under running cold water, then pat dry with paper towels.
3. Transfer the sticks in a large bowl and drizzle with vegetable oil. Toss to coat well. Place the potato sticks in the air fryer basket.
4. Put the air fryer basket on the baking pan and slide into Rack Position 2, select Air Fry, set temperature to 400ºF (205ºC) and set time to 25 minutes.
5. Stir the potato sticks at least three times during cooking.
6. Meanwhile, make the gravy: Heat the butter in a saucepan over medium heat until melted.
7. Add the onion, thyme, and garlic and sauté for 5 minutes or until the onion is translucent.
8. Add the flour and sauté for an additional 2 minutes. Pour in the tomato paste and beef stock and cook for 1 more minute or until lightly thickened.
9. Drizzle the gravy with Worcestershire sauce and sprinkle with salt and ground black pepper. Reduce the heat to low to keep the gravy warm until ready to serve.
10. When done, the sticks should be golden brown. Remove from the oven. Transfer the fried potato sticks onto a plate, then sprinkle with salt and ground black pepper. Scatter with string cheese and pour the gravy over. Serve warm.

482.Asian Dipping Sauce

Servings: About 1 Cup
Cooking Time: 0 Minutes
Ingredients:
- ¼ cup rice vinegar
- ¼ cup hoisin sauce
- ¼ cup low-sodium chicken or vegetable stock
- 3 tablespoons soy sauce
- 1 tablespoon minced or grated ginger
- 1 tablespoon minced or pressed garlic
- 1 teaspoon chili-garlic sauce or sriracha (or more to taste)

Directions:
1. Stir together all the ingredients in a small bowl, or place in a jar with a tight-fitting lid and shake until well mixed.
2. Use immediately.

483.Simple Teriyaki Sauce

Servings: ¾ Cup
Cooking Time: 0 Minutes
Ingredients:
- ½ cup soy sauce
- 3 tablespoons honey
- 1 tablespoon rice wine or dry sherry
- 1 tablespoon rice vinegar
- 2 teaspoons minced fresh ginger
- 2 garlic cloves, smashed

Directions:
1. Beat together all the ingredients in a small bowl.
2. Use immediately.

484.Fast Cinnamon Toast

Servings: 6
Cooking Time: 5 Minutes
Ingredients:
- 1½ teaspoons cinnamon
- 1½ teaspoons vanilla extract
- ½ cup sugar
- 2 teaspoons ground black pepper
- 2 tablespoons melted coconut oil
- 12 slices whole wheat bread

Directions:
1. Combine all the ingredients, except for the bread, in a large bowl. Stir to mix well.
2. Dunk the bread in the bowl of mixture gently to coat and infuse well. Shake the excess off. Arrange the bread slices in the air fryer basket.

3. Put the air fryer basket on the baking pan and slide into Rack Position 2, select Air Fry, set temperature to 400ºF (205ºC) and set time to 5 minutes.
4. Flip the bread halfway through.
5. When cooking is complete, the bread should be golden brown.
6. Remove the bread slices from the oven and slice to serve.

485.Chocolate And Coconut Macaroons

Servings: 24 Macaroons
Cooking Time: 8 Minutes
Ingredients:
- 3 large egg whites, at room temperature
- ¼ teaspoon salt
- ¾ cup granulated white sugar
- 4½ tablespoons unsweetened cocoa powder
- 2¼ cups unsweetened shredded coconut

Directions:
1. Line the air fryer basket with parchment paper.
2. Whisk the egg whites with salt in a large bowl with a hand mixer on high speed until stiff peaks form.
3. Whisk in the sugar with the hand mixer on high speed until the mixture is thick. Mix in the cocoa powder and coconut.
4. Scoop 2 tablespoons of the mixture and shape the mixture in a ball. Repeat with remaining mixture to make 24 balls in total.
5. Arrange the balls in a single layer in the basket and leave a little space between each two balls.
6. Put the air fryer basket on the baking pan and slide into Rack Position 2, select Air Fry, set temperature to 375ºF (190ºC) and set time to 8 minutes.
7. When cooking is complete, the balls should be golden brown.
8. Serve immediately.

486.Pastrami Casserole

Servings: 2
Cooking Time: 8 Minutes
Ingredients:
- 1 cup pastrami, sliced
- 1 bell pepper, chopped
- ¼ cup Greek yogurt
- 2 spring onions, chopped
- ½ cup Cheddar cheese, grated
- 4 eggs
- ¼ teaspoon ground black pepper
- Sea salt, to taste
- Cooking spray

Directions:
1. Spritz the baking pan with cooking spray.
2. Whisk together all the ingredients in a large bowl. Stir to mix well. Pour the mixture into the baking pan.
3. Slide the baking pan into Rack Position 1, select Convection Bake, set temperature to 330ºF (166ºC) and set time to 8 minutes.
4. When cooking is complete, the eggs should be set and the casserole edges should be lightly browned.
5. Remove from the oven and allow to cool for 10 minutes before serving.

487.Garlicky Olive Stromboli

Servings: 8
Cooking Time: 25 Minutes
Ingredients:
- 4 large cloves garlic, unpeeled
- 3 tablespoons grated Parmesan cheese
- ½ cup packed fresh basil leaves
- ½ cup marinated, pitted green and black olives
- ¼ teaspoon crushed red pepper
- ½ pound (227 g) pizza dough, at room temperature
- 4 ounces (113 g) sliced provolone cheese (about 8 slices)
- Cooking spray

Directions:
1. Spritz the air fryer basket with cooking spray. Put the unpeeled garlic in the basket.
2. Put the air fryer basket on the baking pan and slide into Rack Position 2, select Air Fry, set temperature to 370ºF (188ºC) and set time to 10 minutes.
3. When cooked, the garlic will be softened completely. Remove from the oven and allow to cool until you can handle.
4. Peel the garlic and place into a food processor with 2 tablespoons of Parmesan, basil, olives, and crushed red pepper. Pulse to mix well. Set aside.
5. Arrange the pizza dough on a clean work surface, then roll it out with a rolling pin into a rectangle. Cut the rectangle in half.
6. Sprinkle half of the garlic mixture over each rectangle half, and leave ½-inch edges uncover. Top them with the provolone cheese.
7. Brush one long side of each rectangle half with water, then roll them up. Spritz the basket with cooking spray. Transfer the rolls to the basket. Spritz with cooking spray and scatter with remaining Parmesan.
8. Select Air Fry and set time to 15 minutes.
9. Flip the rolls halfway through the cooking time. When done, the rolls should be golden brown.

10. Remove the rolls from the oven and allow to cool for a few minutes before serving.

488.Classic Churros

Servings: 12 Churros
Cooking Time: 10 Minutes
Ingredients:
- 4 tablespoons butter
- ¼ teaspoon salt
- ½ cup water
- ½ cup all-purpose flour
- 2 large eggs
- 2 teaspoons ground cinnamon
- ¼ cup granulated white sugar
- Cooking spray

Directions:
1. Put the butter, salt, and water in a saucepan. Bring to a boil until the butter is melted on high heat. Keep stirring.
2. Reduce the heat to medium and fold in the flour to form a dough. Keep cooking and stirring until the dough is dried out and coat the pan with a crust.
3. Turn off the heat and scrape the dough in a large bowl. Allow to cool for 15 minutes.
4. Break and whisk the eggs into the dough with a hand mixer until the dough is sanity and firm enough to shape.
5. Scoop up 1 tablespoon of the dough and roll it into a ½-inch-diameter and 2-inch-long cylinder. Repeat with remaining dough to make 12 cylinders in total.
6. Combine the cinnamon and sugar in a large bowl and dunk the cylinders into the cinnamon mix to coat.
7. Arrange the cylinders on a plate and refrigerate for 20 minutes.
8. Spritz the air fryer basket with cooking spray. Place the cylinders in the basket and spritz with cooking spray.
9. Put the air fryer basket on the baking pan and slide into Rack Position 2, select Air Fry, set temperature to 375ºF (190ºC) and set time to 10 minutes.
10. Flip the cylinders halfway through the cooking time.
11. When cooked, the cylinders should be golden brown and fluffy.
12. Serve immediately.

489.Bartlett Pears With Lemony Ricotta

Servings: 4
Cooking Time: 8 Minutes
Ingredients:
- 2 large Bartlett pears, peeled, cut in half, cored

- 3 tablespoons melted butter
- ½ teaspoon ground ginger
- ¼ teaspoon ground cardamom
- 3 tablespoons brown sugar
- ½ cup whole-milk ricotta cheese
- 1 teaspoon pure lemon extract
- 1 teaspoon pure almond extract
- 1 tablespoon honey, plus additional for drizzling

Directions:
1. Toss the pears with butter, ginger, cardamom, and sugar in a large bowl. Toss to coat well. Arrange the pears in the baking pan, cut side down.
2. Put the air fryer basket on the baking pan and slide into Rack Position 2, select Air Fry, set temperature to 375ºF (190ºC) and set time to 8 minutes.
3. After 5 minutes, remove the pan and flip the pears. Return to the oven and continue cooking.
4. When cooking is complete, the pears should be soft and browned. Remove from the oven.
5. In the meantime, combine the remaining ingredients in a separate bowl. Whip for 1 minute with a hand mixer until the mixture is puffed.
6. Divide the mixture into four bowls, then put the pears over the mixture and drizzle with more honey to serve.

490.Parsnip Fries With Garlic-yogurt Dip

Servings: 4
Cooking Time: 10 Minutes
Ingredients:
- 3 medium parsnips, peeled, cut into sticks
- ¼ teaspoon kosher salt
- 1 teaspoon olive oil
- 1 garlic clove, unpeeled
- Cooking spray
- Dip:
- ¼ cup plain Greek yogurt
- ⅛ teaspoon garlic powder
- 1 tablespoon sour cream
- ¼ teaspoon kosher salt
- Freshly ground black pepper, to taste

Directions:
1. Spritz the air fryer basket with cooking spray.
2. Put the parsnip sticks in a large bowl, then sprinkle with salt and drizzle with olive oil.
3. Transfer the parsnip into the basket and add the garlic.
4. Put the air fryer basket on the baking pan and slide into Rack Position 2, select Air Fry, set temperature to 360ºF (182ºC) and set time to 10 minutes.
5. Stir the parsnip halfway through the cooking time.

6. Meanwhile, peel the garlic and crush it. Combine the crushed garlic with the ingredients for the dip. Stir to mix well.
7. When cooked, the parsnip sticks should be crisp. Remove the parsnip fries from the oven and serve with the dipping sauce.

491.Pão De Queijo

Servings: 12 Balls
Cooking Time: 12 Minutes
Ingredients:
- 2 tablespoons butter, plus more for greasing
- ½ cup milk
- 1½ cups tapioca flour
- ½ teaspoon salt
- 1 large egg
- ²/₃ cup finely grated aged Asiago cheese

Directions:
1. Put the butter in a saucepan and pour in the milk, heat over medium heat until the liquid boils. Keep stirring.
2. Turn off the heat and mix in the tapioca flour and salt to form a soft dough. Transfer the dough in a large bowl, then wrap the bowl in plastic and let sit for 15 minutes.
3. Break the egg in the bowl of dough and whisk with a hand mixer for 2 minutes or until a sanity dough forms. Fold the cheese in the dough. Cover the bowl in plastic again and let sit for 10 more minutes.
4. Grease the baking pan with butter.
5. Scoop 2 tablespoons of the dough into the baking pan. Repeat with the remaining dough to make dough 12 balls. Keep a little distance between each two balls.
6. Slide the baking pan into Rack Position 1, select Convection Bake, set temperature to 375ºF (190ºC) and set time to 12 minutes.
7. Flip the balls halfway through the cooking time.
8. When cooking is complete, the balls should be golden brown and fluffy.
9. Remove the balls from the oven and allow to cool for 5 minutes before serving.

492.Sausage And Colorful Peppers Casserole

Servings: 6
Cooking Time: 25 Minutes
Ingredients:
- 1 pound (454 g) minced breakfast sausage
- 1 yellow pepper, diced
- 1 red pepper, diced
- 1 green pepper, diced
- 1 sweet onion, diced
- 2 cups Cheddar cheese, shredded
- 6 eggs
- Salt and freshly ground black pepper, to taste
- Fresh parsley, for garnish

Directions:
1. Cook the sausage in a nonstick skillet over medium heat for 10 minutes or until well browned. Stir constantly.
2. When the cooking is finished, transfer the cooked sausage to the baking pan and add the peppers and onion. Scatter with Cheddar cheese.
3. Whisk the eggs with salt and ground black pepper in a large bowl, then pour the mixture into the baking pan.
4. Slide the baking pan into Rack Position 1, select Convection Bake, set temperature to 360ºF (182ºC) and set time to 15 minutes.
5. When cooking is complete, the egg should be set and the edges of the casserole should be lightly browned.
6. Remove from the oven and top with fresh parsley before serving.

493.Cheesy Green Bean Casserole

Servings: 4
Cooking Time: 6 Minutes
Ingredients:
- 1 tablespoon melted butter
- 1 cup green beans
- 6 ounces (170 g) Cheddar cheese, shredded
- 7 ounces (198 g) Parmesan cheese, shredded
- ¼ cup heavy cream
- Sea salt, to taste

Directions:
1. Grease the baking pan with the melted butter.
2. Add the green beans, Cheddar, salt, and black pepper to the prepared baking pan. Stir to mix well, then spread the Parmesan and cream on top.
3. Slide the baking pan into Rack Position 1, select Convection Bake, set temperature to 400ºF (205ºC) and set time to 6 minutes.
4. When cooking is complete, the beans should be tender and the cheese should be melted.
5. Serve immediately.

494.Sweet And Sour Peanuts

Servings: 9
Cooking Time: 5 Minutes
Ingredients:
- 3 cups shelled raw peanuts
- 1 tablespoon hot red pepper sauce
- 3 tablespoons granulated white sugar

Directions:

1. Put the peanuts in a large bowl, then drizzle with hot red pepper sauce and sprinkle with sugar. Toss to coat well.
2. Pour the peanuts in the air fryer basket.
3. Put the air fryer basket on the baking pan and slide into Rack Position 2, select Air Fry, set temperature to 400ºF (205ºC) and set time to 5 minutes.
4. Stir the peanuts halfway through the cooking time.
5. When cooking is complete, the peanuts will be crispy and browned. Remove from the oven and serve immediately.

495.South Carolina Shrimp And Corn Bake

Servings: 2
Cooking Time: 18 Minutes
Ingredients:
- 1 ear corn, husk and silk removed, cut into 2-inch rounds
- 8 ounces (227 g) red potatoes, unpeeled, cut into 1-inch pieces
- 2 teaspoons Old Bay Seasoning, divided
- 2 teaspoons vegetable oil, divided
- ¼ teaspoon ground black pepper
- 8 ounces (227 g) large shrimps (about 12 shrimps), deveined
- 6 ounces (170 g) andouille or chorizo sausage, cut into 1-inch pieces
- 2 garlic cloves, minced
- 1 tablespoon chopped fresh parsley
Directions:
1. Put the corn rounds and potatoes in a large bowl. Sprinkle with 1 teaspoon of Old Bay seasoning and drizzle with vegetable oil. Toss to coat well.
2. Transfer the corn rounds and potatoes into the baking pan.
3. Slide the baking pan into Rack Position 1, select Convection Bake, set temperature to 400ºF (205ºC) and set time to 18 minutes.
4. After 6 minutes, remove from the oven. Stir the corn rounds and potatoes. Return the pan to the oven and continue cooking.
5. Meanwhile, cut slits into the shrimps but be careful not to cut them through. Combine the shrimps, sausage, remaining Old Bay seasoning, and remaining vegetable oil in the large bowl. Toss to coat well.
6. After 6 minutes, remove the pan from the oven. Add the shrimps and sausage to the pan. Return the pan to the oven and continue cooking for 6 minutes. Stir the shrimp mixture halfway through the cooking time.

7. When done, the shrimps should be opaque. Transfer the dish to a plate and spread with parsley before serving.

496.Butternut Squash With Hazelnuts

Servings: 3 Cups
Cooking Time: 23 Minutes
Ingredients:
- 2 tablespoons whole hazelnuts
- 3 cups butternut squash, peeled, deseeded and cubed
- ¼ teaspoon kosher salt
- ¼ teaspoon freshly ground black pepper
- 2 teaspoons olive oil
- Cooking spray
Directions:
1. Spritz the air fryer basket with cooking spray. Spread the hazelnuts in the pan.
2. Put the air fryer basket on the baking pan and slide into Rack Position 2, select Air Fry, set temperature to 300ºF (150ºC) and set time to 3 minutes.
3. When done, the hazelnuts should be soft. Remove from the oven. Chopped the hazelnuts roughly and transfer to a small bowl. Set aside.
4. Put the butternut squash in a large bowl, then sprinkle with salt and pepper and drizzle with olive oil. Toss to coat well. Transfer the squash to the lightly greased basket.
5. Put the air fryer basket on the baking pan and slide into Rack Position 2, select Air Fry, set temperature to 360ºF (182ºC) and set time to 20 minutes.
6. Flip the squash halfway through the cooking time.
7. When cooking is complete, the squash will be soft. Transfer the squash to a plate and sprinkle with the chopped hazelnuts before serving.

497.Spinach And Chickpea Casserole

Servings: 4
Cooking Time: 21 To 22 Minutes
Ingredients:
- 2 tablespoons olive oil
- 2 garlic cloves, minced
- 1 tablespoon ginger, minced
- 1 onion, chopped
- 1 chili pepper, minced
- Salt and ground black pepper, to taste
- 1 pound (454 g) spinach
- 1 can coconut milk
- ½ cup dried tomatoes, chopped
- 1 (14-ounce / 397-g) can chickpeas, drained

Directions:
1. Heat the olive oil in a saucepan over medium heat. Sauté the garlic and ginger in the olive oil for 1 minute, or until fragrant.
2. Add the onion, chili pepper, salt and pepper to the saucepan. Sauté for 3 minutes.
3. Mix in the spinach and sauté for 3 to 4 minutes or until the vegetables become soft. Remove from heat.
4. Pour the vegetable mixture into the baking pan. Stir in coconut milk, dried tomatoes and chickpeas until well blended.
5. Slide the baking pan into Rack Position 1, select Convection Bake, set temperature to 370ºF (188ºC) and set time to 15 minutes.
6. When cooking is complete, transfer the casserole to a serving dish. Let cool for 5 minutes before serving.

498.Chinese Pork And Mushroom Egg Rolls

Servings: 25 Egg Rolls
Cooking Time: 33 Minutes
Ingredients:
- Egg Rolls:
- 1 tablespoon mirin
- 3 tablespoons soy sauce, divided
- 1 pound (454 g) ground pork
- 3 tablespoons vegetable oil, plus more for brushing
- 5 ounces (142 g) shiitake mushrooms, minced
- 4 cups shredded Napa cabbage
- ¼ cup sliced scallions
- 1 teaspoon grated fresh ginger
- 1 clove garlic, minced
- ¼ teaspoon cornstarch
- 1 (1-pound / 454-g) package frozen egg roll wrappers, thawed
- Dipping Sauce:
- 1 scallion, white and light green parts only, sliced
- ¼ cup rice vinegar
- ¼ cup soy sauce
- Pinch sesame seeds
- Pinch red pepper flakes
- 1 teaspoon granulated sugar

Directions:
1. Line the air fryer basket with parchment paper. Set aside.
2. Combine the mirin and 1 tablespoon of soy sauce in a large bowl. Stir to mix well.
3. Dunk the ground pork in the mixture and stir to mix well. Wrap the bowl in plastic and marinate in the refrigerator for at least 10 minutes.

4. Heat the vegetable oil in a nonstick skillet over medium-high heat until shimmering. Add the mushrooms, cabbage, and scallions and sauté for 5 minutes or until tender.
5. Add the marinated meat, ginger, garlic, and remaining 2 tablespoons of soy sauce. Sauté for 3 minutes or until the pork is lightly browned. Turn off the heat and allow to cool until ready to use.
6. Put the cornstarch in a small bowl and pour in enough water to dissolve the cornstarch. Put the bowl alongside a clean work surface.
7. Put the egg roll wrappers in the basket.
8. Put the air fryer basket on the baking pan and slide into Rack Position 2, select Air Fry, set temperature to 400ºF (205ºC) and set time to 15 minutes.
9. Flip the wrappers halfway through the cooking time.
10. When cooked, the wrappers will be golden brown. Remove the egg roll wrappers from the oven and allow to cool for 10 minutes or until you can handle them with your hands.
11. Lay out one egg roll wrapper on the work surface with a corner pointed toward you. Place 2 tablespoons of the pork mixture on the egg roll wrapper and fold corner up over the mixture. Fold left and right corners toward the center and continue to roll. Brush a bit of the dissolved cornstarch on the last corner to help seal the egg wrapper. Repeat with remaining wrappers to make 25 egg rolls in total.
12. Arrange the rolls in the basket and brush the rolls with more vegetable oil.
13. Select Air Fry and set time to 10 minutes. Return to the oven. When done, the rolls should be well browned and crispy.
14. Meanwhile, combine the ingredients for the dipping sauce in a small bowl. Stir to mix well.
15. Serve the rolls with the dipping sauce immediately.

499.Roasted Mushrooms

Servings: About 1½ Cups
Cooking Time: 30 Minutes
Ingredients:
- 1 pound (454 g) button or cremini mushrooms, washed, stems trimmed, and cut into quarters or thick slices
- ¼ cup water
- 1 teaspoon kosher salt or ½ teaspoon fine salt
- 3 tablespoons unsalted butter, cut into pieces, or extra-virgin olive oil

Directions:
1. Place a large piece of aluminum foil on the sheet pan. Place the mushroom pieces in the middle of the foil. Spread them out into an even layer. Pour the

water over them, season with the salt, and add the butter. Wrap the mushrooms in the foil.
2.   Select Roast, set the temperature to 325ºF (163ºC), and set the time for 15 minutes. Select Start to begin preheating.
3.   Once the unit has preheated, place the pan in the oven.
4.   After 15 minutes, remove the pan from the oven. Transfer the foil packet to a cutting board and carefully unwrap it. Pour the mushrooms and cooking liquid from the foil onto the sheet pan.
5.   Select Roast, set the temperature to 350ºF (180ºC), and set the time for 15 minutes. Return the pan to the oven. Select Start to begin.
6.   After about 10 minutes, remove the pan from the oven and stir the mushrooms. Return the pan to the oven and continue cooking for anywhere from 5 to 15 more minutes, or until the liquid is mostly gone and the mushrooms start to brown.
7.   Serve immediately.

500.Keto Cheese Quiche

Servings: 8
Cooking Time: 1 Hour
Ingredients:
- Crust:
- 1¼ cups blanched almond flour
- 1 large egg, beaten
- 1¼ cups grated Parmesan cheese
- ¼ teaspoon fine sea salt
- Filling:
- 4 ounces (113 g) cream cheese
- 1 cup shredded Swiss cheese
- $^1/_3$ cup minced leeks
- 4 large eggs, beaten
- ½ cup chicken broth
- ⅛ teaspoon cayenne pepper
- ¾ teaspoon fine sea salt
- 1 tablespoon unsalted butter, melted
- Chopped green onions, for garnish
- Cooking spray

Directions:
1.   Spritz the baking pan with cooking spray.
2.   Combine the flour, egg, Parmesan, and salt in a large bowl. Stir to mix until a satiny and firm dough forms.
3.   Arrange the dough between two grease parchment papers, then roll the dough into a $^1/_{16}$-inch thick circle.
4.   Make the crust: Transfer the dough into the prepared pan and press to coat the bottom.
5.   Slide the baking pan into Rack Position 1, select Convection Bake, set temperature to 325ºF (163ºC) and set time to 12 minutes.
6.   When cooking is complete, the edges of the crust should be lightly browned.
7.   Meanwhile, combine the ingredient for the filling, except for the green onions in a large bowl.
8.   Pour the filling over the cooked crust and cover the edges of the crust with aluminum foil.
9.   Slide the baking pan into Rack Position 1, select Convection Bake, set time to 15 minutes.
10.   When cooking is complete, reduce the heat to 300ºF (150ºC) and set time to 30 minutes.
11.   When cooking is complete, a toothpick inserted in the center should come out clean.
12.   Remove from the oven and allow to cool for 10 minutes before serving.

CPSIA information can be obtained
at www.ICGtesting.com
Printed in the USA
LVHW101622190521
687904LV00011B/447

9 781801 663335